Collagen
HANDBOOK

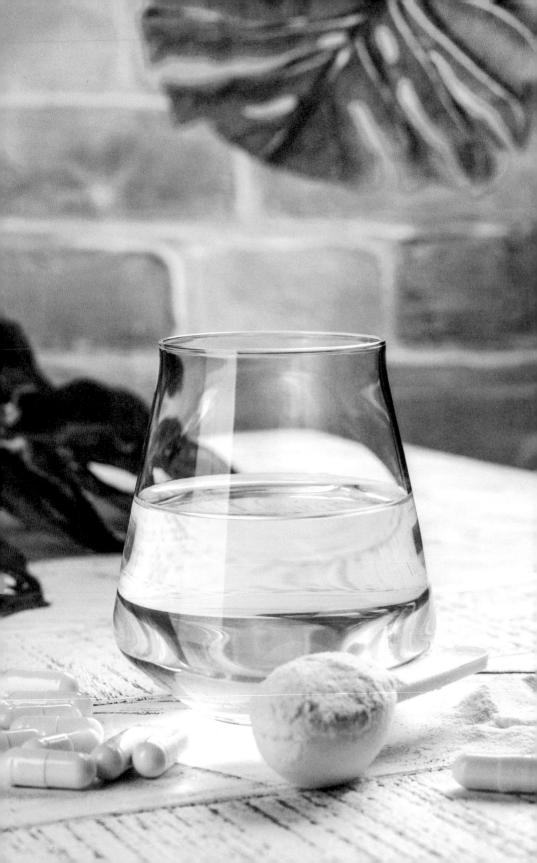

Recipes for Natural Living

Collagen

HANDBOOK

KIMBERLY HOLLAND

Foreword by Carolyn Williams, PhD, RD

STERLING
New York

STERLING
New York

An Imprint of Sterling Publishing Co., Inc.
1166 Avenue of the Americas
New York, NY 10036

ISBN 978-1-4549-3661-9

Distributed in Canada by Sterling Publishing Co., Inc.
c/o Canadian Manda Group, 664 Annette Street
Toronto, Ontario M6S 2C8, Canada
Distributed in the United Kingdom by GMC Distribution Services
Castle Place, 166 High Street, Lewes, East Sussex BN7 1XU, England
Distributed in Australia by NewSouth Books
University of New South Wales, Sydney, NSW 2052, Australia

For information about custom editions, special sales,
and premium and corporate purchases, please
contact Sterling Special Sales at 800-805-5489
or specialsales@sterlingpublishing.com.

Manufactured in Canada

2 4 6 8 10 9 7 5 3 1

sterlingpublishing.com

Cover design by Elizabeth Mihaltse Lindy
Interior design by Christine Heun

For image credits - see page 162

For my mom,
who never fails to believe in me.

CONTENTS

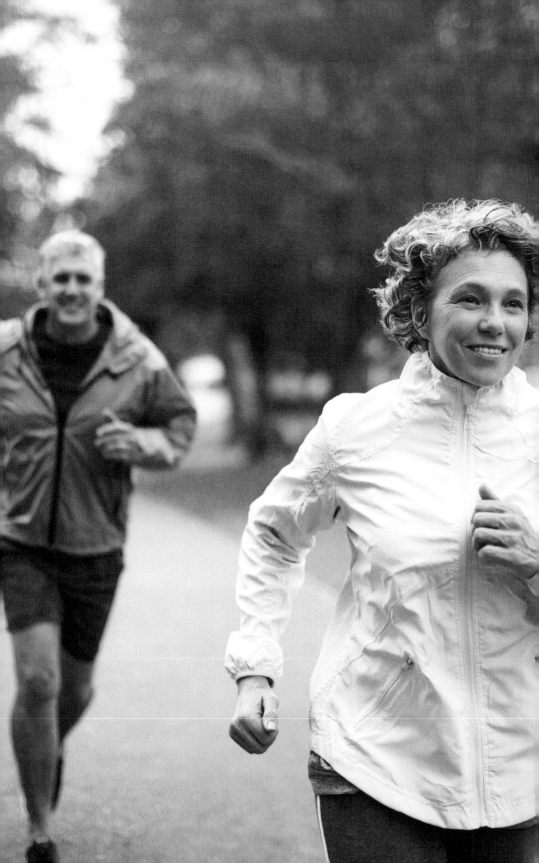

FOREWORD

I t was a charismatic anatomy professor who first piqued my interest in the health field, which ultimately led to my now more than twenty-year career as a registered dietitian. She brought to life just how amazingly orchestrated, adaptive, and resilient the human body is designed to be, and she made complicated physiology understandable—even fascinating—by regularly challenging us to compare the body to a car or other motorized machines. As she explained, the body is constantly "on," or running, keeping the heart beating, blood pumping, lungs breathing, hormones secreted, and so on. As anything running nonstop requires proper maintenance and care to stay operating effectively and efficiently, in the body's case, this includes habits like eating a healthy diet with adequate nutrients, getting regular activity, and reducing stress.

Because of that professor, most of my work has been spent teaching others how to best use food and nutrients to enhance the running of their bodies to meet health goals. And I regularly use her car analogy, and the importance of the car's maintenance, to help others see how the nutrients and compounds they consume affect overall health, wellness, and the aging process. Granted, genetics plays a large role in how efficiently each body runs and responds, but there are certain nutrients and compounds that can either interfere with or enhance how we all run. For decades, however, the emphasis, from a nutrition perspective, has been primarily placed on those with negative effects—the known harmful nutrients like sodium, added sugar, trans fats, and other compounds that we need to avoid. In fact, the idea that the nutrients and compounds you consume can be used proactively to have tangible health benefits—and maybe even antiaging effects—was largely dismissed by most health professionals for years. It was seen as more important to focus on avoiding the "bad" ones.

Today, thanks to a multitude of studies over the past ten to fifteen years that have delved into understanding the aging process as part of overall health, the role that diet may play in the body's maintenance and the aging process of the body's systems and tissues has slowly shifted. Our knowledge has increased when it comes to dietary compounds that have great potential to enhance how our body functions, and a key one is collagen. As author Kimberly Holland explains, collagen is the body's internal "glue." It supports soft tissue, reduces inflammation, and speeds up the repair of damaged cells. In fact, collagen is in almost every type of tissue in the body, including bones, muscles, skin, ligaments, tendons, cartilage, artery walls, teeth, and scar tissue. And, during the first thirty years of life, the body does a pretty good job when it comes to making enough collagen to support all its uses. After that, production gradually slows. This explains why many initial signs of aging or wear and tear don't start to show up until after age thirty or forty. And it also explains why there is such interest in how we might support existing collagen and promote production through dietary means.

The idea that extra collagen in the body might be able to slow, or even reverse, the aging process has catapulted it into the spotlight over the past few years, and it's made *collagen* a trendy buzzword in markets for both antiaging and wellness products. But the media hype and publicity surrounding products containing the natural compound have also made finding accurate information difficult. In addition, while there are some food sources for collagen, dietary supplements are often a much more plentiful and convenient source. This factor can add to consumer confusion since the dietary supplement market now includes more than eighty thousand products and there is minimal oversight of these products by the Federal Drug Administration (FDA). The result is that it's more incumbent than ever on consumers to do their research to determine which, if any, products may be beneficial for their needs and which manufacturers can boast reputable products.

This is also exactly why I've found the information in this book to be an invaluable resource when it comes to understanding collagen's potential and how to incorporate it into your lifestyle. With her years of experience working as a journalist in the areas of nutrition and health, Kimberly provides a simple, research-based explanation of what collagen is, the types of collagen in the body, their role in the body, and the various types available from food and supplements and what's on the market. She also presents an unbiased look at the latest in collagen research when it comes not only to skin and appearance but also to joint, bone, muscle, and heart health.

I consider this book an essential reference for anyone even remotely interested or intrigued by collagen's possibilities. It's become my go-to source, and I think it should be yours, too. Just like my long-ago professor's car, anything running nonstop will gradually have a little wear and tear. However, regular maintenance—a part of which may include collagen—can slow the signs of aging and improve overall wellness.

In health,

CAROLYN WILLIAMS, PhD, RD
Registered Dietitian, Culinary Nutrition
Expert, and Author of *Meals That Heal*

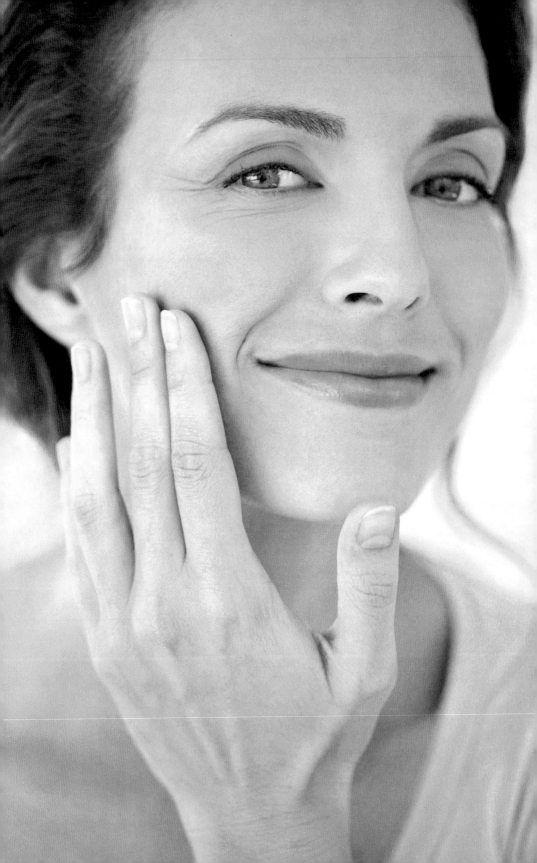

PART 1

All About Collagen

You would not be alone if your primary reference for collagen is cosmetics and, perhaps, fillers for the face. Indeed, for many years, the word *collagen* was most closely associated with the beauty industry and age-erasing injectables.

But today, collagen is bubbling up in many nutrition circles for its possible benefits to everything from, yes, skin, to your joints, bones, gut, and heart. Shelves in grocery stores and health-food chains are filled with collagen supplements. Your friends may even be stirring packets of collagen into their morning coffee. All of this could leave you wondering whether there's any reason you should consider including collagen as part of your diet. Well, the answer is likely yes—and for several good reasons.

Collagen is the most abundant structural protein in the human body. In fact, it makes up 30 percent of all the human body's total protein. It's also the most abundant protein in many animals, which is why beef, chicken, pork, fish, and seafood are some of the best dietary sources of collagen.

Collagen also happens to be a major component of nearly every type of tissue in your body, including muscles, skin, ligaments, tendons, organs, and even your brain. It gives them strength, elasticity, and durability. It connects soft tissues to your skeleton. Collagen provides the cells that make up many of these important components, and it also creates an internal structure to support them.

In short, collagen is everywhere in the body and in almost every body system.

For a period of time, your body can make the collagen it needs, but its production quantity does eventually slow. In your late twenties or early thirties, collagen production begins to fall off, which means the body gradually makes less of the protein than it needs to supply all the necessary functions it performs.

That's when visible signs of aging appear—fine lines, wrinkles, thinning skin—as well as the not-so visible, from achy joints to burgeoning osteoarthritis.

Other lifestyle factors, including sun exposure, poor diet, and alcohol consumption, can further dismantle your natural collagen stores and slow the pace of collagen production.

Collagen loss is natural, as is the slowing collagen production that comes with age, but replacing the collagen could help ease some of these signs of aging and even prevent collagen-related health conditions. Though the research is still in its early years, scientists and doctors have been able to identify key areas in which supplementing your natural collagen is particularly effective.

WHAT'S IN COLLAGEN?

Collagen is composed of a series of amino acids, including arginine, glutamine, glycine, and proline. Among other uses, amino acids are the building blocks for proteins and are essential to synthesizing hormones and transporting chemical messages through the body.

As for collagen, amino acids bind together to form procollagen, a precursor for the protein that's still strong enough to provide strength and structure. To become collagen, procollagen undergoes a grouping process, forming long collagen chains with more than one thousand amino acids. Those chains arrange themselves side by side and bind together into fibrils, or three-dimensional helices.

Many of the unique capabilities of collagen—for example, being elastic and forgiving enough to be stretched without tearing—are thanks to the unique properties of these triple helices. They bind closely together to form a dense sheath of cells and act as the foundation of body materials, whether it's in your epidermis (upper layer of skin), your gut, or anywhere else.

WHAT'S MADE FROM COLLAGEN?

The word *collagen* is derived from the Greek word *kólla*, which means "glue," and the French word *-gène*, which means "something that produces." Glue is exactly what collagen is and what it does to your body's cells, skeleton, and internal organs—it holds everything together.

Groups of collagen fibrils bind, side by side, in dense sheets or fibers. These are the foundation of tissues that make up organs, including your skin. Collagen also is a foundational element of bones, when combined with minerals. It even makes up the majority of tendons and cartilage, the tissues that connect bones and protect the ends of bones from damage and force.

Nails, hair, and teeth are all partly composed of collagen. Muscles, too, are made with collagen, though to a lesser extent than other body materials.

Collagen is also a major component of your body's extracellular matrix.

This three-dimensional network of cells, enzymes, fibers, and collagen provides the structural support necessary for your body to form organs and tissues.

A second matrix then supports all the elements of your body, including those organs and tissues, in another network of collagen-rich extracellular matrices.

Every element of the extracellular matrix (ECM) works together to keep you upright and moving. The extracellular matrix is to tissues and organs what your skeleton is to bones. It pulls together much of what's needed to make the individual bones, tissues, and organs in your body. Then, another ECM forms to support your bones and tissues and maintain their places in your body.

But if that weren't enough, the ECM has a secondary role: it helps inform cell behavior and sends instructions throughout the body. When the ECM detects a cut or scrape, for example, it can pull molecules toward the wound to help focus your body's efforts on healing. The ECM can call on the vast array of proteins, amino acids, and compounds in the body to perform any number of tasks.

COLLAGEN IS EVERYWHERE	
Body material	**Percentage collagen**
Sclera (white part of the eye)	90%
Tendons	80%
Skin	70–80%
Cartilage	60%
Bones	30%
Muscle	1–10%

WHEN WAS COLLAGEN DISCOVERED?

In the mid-twentieth century, renowned biophysicists and biochemists, including Ada E. Yonath, Linus Pauling, and Francis Harry Compton Crick, realized collagen was the product of a regular, molecular structure—that is, repeating strands of molecules. Indian physicist G. N. Ramachandra is credited with creating the first peptide structure that most accurately proposed the triple-helical structure we know collagen has today. His model, which was proposed in the 1950s, remained the primary working model for collagen for decades.

But it wasn't until 1994 that researchers were able to produce the first high-resolution three-dimensional structure of the triple-helical collagen strand. This confirmed a lot of what scientists believed about collagen but had been unable to confirm. It also opened areas of research that scientists are still investigating today.

HOW DID OUR ANCESTORS GET COLLAGEN?

If we're producing supplements to get our fill of collagen in this century, how did our ancestors get it centuries ago? From food. Whole-animal eating, including hide and ligaments, was not uncommon a millennium ago. It wasn't entirely unheard of even two or three hundred years ago. Humans have moved away from that style of cooking and eating only in the last few centuries. The approach to use only prime cuts of protein leaves many elements of animals unused, though these elements contain many of the most nutritious and beneficial parts.

Luckily, renewed interest in animal butchering, producing less waste, and being conscientious of an animal's full utility has stirred up focus on finding ways to utilize all pieces of animals, including the hide and joints. In a sense, this is the modern American eater's way of returning to our roots." Collagen might be new to us now, but it's a prehistoric source of essential nutrition.

WHAT DESTROYS COLLAGEN?

Your body is capable of making collagen, and it does so quite well through your first few decades of life. But age, lifestyle choices, and environmental factors can actually destroy the collagen you make. These elements may even halt collagen production prematurely. This can lead to faster aging within the body and the appearance of age-related conditions on the outside earlier in life.

Many of these factors are the result of unhealthy choices that damage your entire health and well-being. Bolting them from your life won't just protect your skin and collagen, it could also cut your risk for any number of related conditions and problems.

Poor Diet

In order for your body to make collagen efficiently, it relies on a tightly choreographed sequence of events—events that all require participation from other nutrients, amino acids, and hormones. If your diet is low on essential vitamins and minerals, specifically vitamin C, then your body may not be able to produce the collagen it needs. Nutritional deficiencies can lead to low collagen levels and premature aging. A diet that is high in sugar and processed foods puts you at risk for these deficiencies, too.

Sun Exposure

The sun is no friend to collagen. (To be perfectly honest, the sun is no friend to your skin at all.) Ultraviolet (UV) radiation destroys collagen, and research suggests radiation from the sun can also destroy the procollagen building blocks that are present in the skin's layers. Over time, chronic UV exposure can reduce total collagen amounts, cause skin-rebuilding errors, and result in wrinkle formation and eventually a leathery appearance.

Excessive Alcohol Consumption

Like a poor diet, high alcohol consumption can deplete your body of the essential nutrients it needs in order to support collagen production and maintain healthy collagen. If you regularly consume high doses of alcohol, you may find that signs of aging appear faster, as collagen and elastin in your skin are destroyed and not replaced.

It's unclear what effects regular moderate levels of alcohol consumption have. (A moderate level is considered up to one drink per day for most women and up to two drinks per day for most men.)

WHAT'S IN A DRINK?

The National Institutes of Health classifies drinks according to what percentage of alcohol they contain.

Type of alcohol	Total ounces	Percent alcohol
Beer	12 ounces	5%
Wine	5 ounces	12%
Distilled spirits	1.5 ounces	40%

Smoking

Narrowed, constricted blood vessels are one of the side effects of smoking tobacco products. When the blood vessels in your skin cannot move blood, oxygen, and nutrients into the skin, damage starts to show as wrinkles, thinning skin, and discoloration. What's more, many of the thousands of chemicals in tobacco smoke are known to damage collagen and elastin, two of the most prominent fibers in skin. As they're destroyed, your skin's strength and elasticity begin to weaken.

Fast Facts

The importance and role of collagen comes down to these four vital points:

1. Collagen is the most abundant protein in the body. It's used to make a great deal of the body's tissues, muscles, and bones.

2. Collagen is also the glue that holds together many parts of your internal body. Collagen both (1) forms the extracellular matrix (ECM), which binds cells and strands of molecules together to form organs, bones, and tissues, and (2) forms a three-dimensional network that keeps these body elements in place.

3. Collagen is a bit of a train conductor. It can manage cells, regulating where things go when they're needed. For example, collagen can reduce inflammation and speed up the repair of damaged cells from an injury by harnessing the power of cells together.

4. Lastly, collagen is naturally abundant, and the body can use the protein's amino acids to make more collagen. However, by around age thirty, your body will begin making less and less collagen. That's when visible signs of aging may appear. Collagen supplementation can replace much of the lost collagen, which could slow aging and reduce signs and symptoms of some age-related conditions.

TYPES OF COLLAGEN

Given how many roles as collagen plays in the body, from forming the whites of the eyes to connecting soft tissues to bones, it stands to reason that one type of collagen might not be enough. Indeed, several types of collagen are needed. While they may have a lot of similar characteristics—such as being extra flexible and capable of absorbing great resistance—the collagen molecules and strands in your body are not all identical. At least twenty-eight types of collagen exist, and three make up the vast majority of collagen in the human body.

When investigating how collagen works, researchers realized all collagens are made into three-stranded helical segments that are built with side-by-side interactions and bonds. This formation is perhaps in part why collagen has the capacity it does to help muscles, ligaments, and tendons bend and absorb shock but never break.

What separates the many types of collagen, at least on a microscopic level, is how fibers are organized within each helix as well as the arrangement of compounds or amino acids within the fibers.

Proline and glycine are the predominant amino acids in collagen. They're considered nonessential, or conditional, amino acids because your body can make some of its own, but don't let the name fool you—they're vital to health. You can get proline and glycine from animal sources like organ meats. Animal meats, the most common source of protein in the Western diet, have very little of these amino acids.

You may see collagen helices referred to as repeating Gly-Pro-X sequences. *Gly* stands for glycine, *Pro* stands for proline, and X equals any number of amino acids that are used to complete the triple helix. In type I collagen, for example, that X is most commonly hydroxyproline. Each strand of collagen has at least three hundred repeats of this Gly-Pro-X chain.

Knowing the type of amino acids that are used to form collagen can help you understand, at least in part, why collagen has such a profound impact on a person's body. Here are five of the most common collagen amino acids and what they do—apart from helping collagen, of course—to benefit your body.

Glycine

This amino acid is the primary amino acid in collagen chains. Indeed, 33 percent of all amino acids in a collagen protein are glycine. And though it is one of the smallest amino acids, it's incredibly powerful. It helps build healthy DNA strands and forms one-third of the amino acids needed to produce *creatine*, a compound that helps muscles grow and boosts energy.

Glycine is also necessary for antioxidant production, and without it, you might not reap the benefits of all the free radical-fighting foods and drinks or supplements you consume. (Free radicals are charged ions that can damage cells and, in some cases, lead to cell overgrowth, which can become cancerous.) Research even suggests glycine may help protect against alcohol-induced liver damage and promote quality sleep.

Proline

Fifteen percent of collagen is made of this imino acid. Yes, technically, proline is an *imino* acid, not an *amino* acid. It's an organic compound that combines imine with carboxyl, whereas an amino acid combines amino with carboxyl. For the sake of brevity and the purpose of understanding collagen, however, these compounds are typically referred to collectively as amino acids.

In addition to being a building block of collagen, proline has protective benefits for blood vessels and cardiovascular health and is linked to improved joint health. In combination with glycine, proline may also help restore collagen production in layers of skin that have been damaged by ultraviolet radiation from the sun.

Hydroxyproline

This amino acid is necessary for collagen stability. Without it, deficiencies and deformities may pop up, which can lead to complicated conditions and diseases. In order to do its job, hydroxyproline needs vitamin C. Levels may fall too low without this resource, which could cause deficiency symptoms, such as joint destruction or degradation.

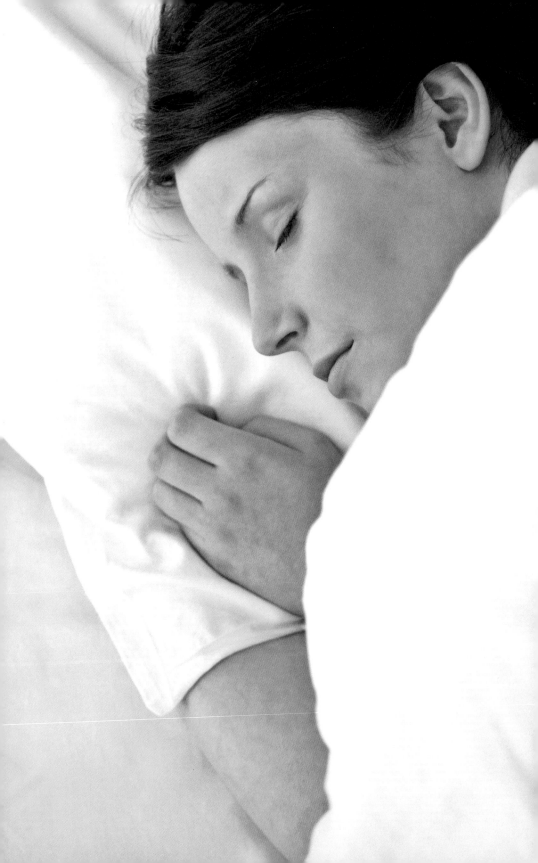

Glutamine

Like proline and glycine, glutamine is an abundant type of amino acid in collagen. In addition to helping generate collagen, this amino acid aids in building muscles and boosting intestinal health. Glutamine helps maintain a barrier between what's on the inside of your intestines and the rest of your body. This can ease symptoms of gastro issues.

Arginine

This amino acid is sometimes written as l-arginine, and it's primarily appreciated for its ability to turn into nitric oxide in the body, which helps expand or dilate blood vessels and reduce blood pressure. Arginine may also improve circulation, improve wound healing, and strengthen the immune system.

THE MAIN TYPES OF COLLAGEN

While there may be more than two dozen identified amino acids, the vast majority of the weight of collagen work in the body is carried by just three: type I, type II, and type III. Type I alone may make up 80 percent of the body's supply of collagen.

> "Gram for gram, type I collagen is stronger than steel," wrote the authors of *Molecular Cell Biology*, fourth edition.

Type I

* **Where it is:** connective tissues, cartilage, skin, bones, tendons, scar tissue, artery walls, teeth, corneas

* **Most notable quality:** makes up at least 80 percent of the collagen in the body

* **Related disease:** Brittle bone disease (bones don't have enough collagen and break easily)

Type I collagen is a primary building block for many of the materials in your body, from teeth and eyes to ligaments and bones. The collagen fibrils and bundled fibers are so plentiful that they not only make up the reinforcement rods of bones, they're also part of the ligaments and tendons that hold those bones in their joints. Type I fibrils are part of the infrastructure that connects soft tissues to bones, too, and they work to replace themselves with new, stronger collagen cells all the time.

Type I collagen is the most abundant type of collagen in the body. Not only does it help form many of the most important materials in the body, it also gives skin its elasticity, or its enormous tensile strength. In other words, collagen helps skin stretch, twist, and bend, but the molecular properties of cartilage (the helices are wrapped so tightly and packed so close together) are such that the collagen doesn't tear.

Because type I collagen is so easy to collect (it's also the most plentiful form in animal products), it's used in many collagen supplements.

WHAT'S BRITTLE BONE DISEASE?

The tight, side-by-side construction of collagen fibrils is what gives the many types of collagen their strength, elasticity, and durability. The specific structural alignments are what determine one type of collagen from another. The arrangement of these strands of amino acids is also what determines whether collagen will perform as it should. Unfortunately, these structural requirements are susceptible to mutation.

In rare instances, genetic mutations prevent the strong-as-steel triple helices of collagen fibrils from forming. This can lead to a condition known as osteogenesis imperfecta, or brittle bone disease. People with this condition have bones that break easily; they may also have bone deformities.

The severity of the condition can vary from person to person. In cases where the disease is mild, a fall and bone break may be the first time a doctor recognizes the bone's inferior construction. In more severe cases, bones may break easily, sometimes even without an accident or use of force. In rare cases, babies born with a particularly severe variation of the condition do not survive long after birth.

To date, there is no cure for brittle bone disease. Treatments largely depend on the severity of the symptoms. Common treatment options include physical therapy, occupational therapy, mobility aids, and surgery. The primary goal of treatment is to prevent fractures. If a fracture does occur, the goal should be to properly treat the break, maintain mobility, and work to strengthen muscles and bones as much as possible.

Type II

* **Where it is:** cartilage

* **Most notable quality:** strength and compressibility

* **Related disease:** chondrodysplasias (abnormal development of cartilage and eventual bone deformities)

Type II collagen is the main component of cartilage, a type of connective tissue. This type of collagen helps joints stay healthy by protecting them from the damage of movement and the compression of weight. When the cartilage in ligaments is healthy because of collagen quantity, the tissue can better resist joint deterioration, joint pain, and potential arthritis.

Some collagen supplement manufacturers make cartilage-specific collagen powder. If you're considering increasing your intake of collagen in order to ease joint pain or symptoms of arthritis, this may be the option you want to consider when purchasing powders.

Type III

* **Where it is:** organs, muscles, arteries, and reticular fibers

* **Most notable quality:** its netlike structure

* **Related disease:** Ehlers-Danlos syndrome, which can lead to deformities in connective tissues or even arteries

A network of fine fibers is the hallmark trait of type III collagen. These reticular (or netlike) fibers form a major portion of the body's extracellular matrix, which is plentiful in bones, ligaments, and tissues throughout the body, as well as in bone marrow. Type III collagen is typically found with type I when in the body because the two work closely together to give skin its firmness and elasticity. This type is known to give blood vessels and tissues in the heart their shape, too.

Type IV

* **Where it is:** basal lamina (layer in the extracellular matrix)

* **Most notable quality:** one part of the basement membrane

Below several layers of skin sit basal lamina, gel-like cushions that separate your upper layers of skin from other structures. This includes your organs and bits of the extracellular matrix around the organs. Type IV collagen is also found in the digestive system and on the surfaces of respiratory elements.

Type V

* **Where it is:** hair and tissue

* **Most notable quality:** also forms the placenta during pregnancy

The fifth type of collagen is necessary to the body's production of cells. Type V collagen makes the surface of cells, which ultimately gives strength to hair and nails. Research suggests this type of collagen is also necessary for expecting mothers, as collagen makes up the primary component of the placenta, an organ that supports a growing fetus.

No matter the type of collagen or the exact arrangement of the structures inside collagen helices, they all serve the same purpose in the body: to strengthen, repair, or help tissues withstand stretching.

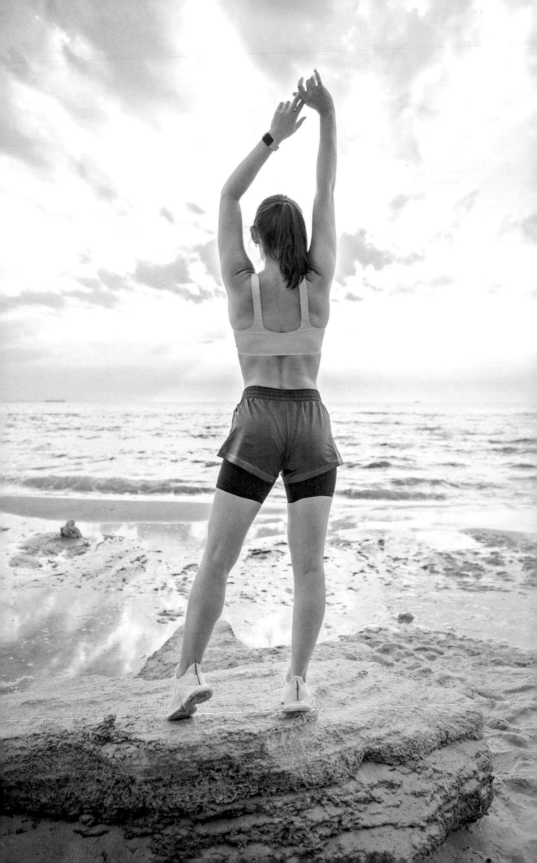

SUPPLEMENTAL SOURCES OF COLLAGEN BY TYPE

Type of supplement	Type of collagen
Beef or bovine collagen supplements	types I and III
Chicken collagen supplements	type II
Eggshell membrane collagen supplements	mostly type I, some III and IV
Fish collagen	type I

Fast Facts

Type I collagen is the most common type of collagen in the body. Indeed, types I, II, and III make up 80 to 90 percent of all the body's collagen. Each type—and there are more than a dozen—has unique roles in the body, and any mutations or damage to the genes of the collagen may result in illnesses or conditions.

THE SOURCES OF COLLAGEN

For the first two to three decades of your life, your body naturally makes a great deal of collagen—at least, as much as you need to maintain healthy skin, protect bones, and guard against some diseases or health conditions. With age, however, collagen production wanes. Despite what you eat or your lifestyle choices, your body just won't make as much collagen as it once did.

But research suggests there are legitimate and beneficial ways to add to the collagen you're losing and stimulate your body into actually producing more collagen. The answer to both is supplementing your diet with collagen, whether that be with food or with processed (hydrolyzed) collagen.

WHAT'S HYDROLYZED COLLAGEN?

Collagen comes from animal sources, like hide, bones, and ligaments. From those elements, manufacturers can produce a type of gelatin that retains all the healthful benefits of collagen but in a more bioavailable form (aka a form that's easier for your body to process). This gelatin can be used in recipes, though it's not as easy to use as collagen peptides, which generally come in powder form.

To make this gelatin collagen easier to cook with and eat, it can be heated and processed to form the collagen supplements you see on store shelves. When the gelatin is heated, the long collagen chains are broken down into shorter ones. These short sections of amino acids are easier for your body to absorb, which means you can reap benefits faster. This processed form of gelatin collagen contains the same amino acids and compounds as the original collagen, but it's ultimately in a form that your body can use more easily.

Research suggests hydrolyzed collagen may be available to your body within an hour of oral ingestion. In fact, one study found that as much as 90 percent of the protein and amino acids were available in that short timeframe. That allows for a speedy and efficient delivery of collagen to various sites in the body.

WHAT ARE COLLAGEN PEPTIDES?

Collagen peptides are another name for hydrolyzed collagen. Some supplement brands will use the word peptides to refer to collagen that comes from animals only, preferring to call collagen from seafood or fish marine collagen. It's a distinction without a difference as far as the chemical makeup is concerned. In this book, *hydrolyzed collagen, collagen hydrolysate, collagen peptides,* and *collagen supplements* are used interchangeably because they are the same thing. It will be noted whenever one type from a particular source makes more sense or has more benefits than another type.

WHY FOOD IS GOOD FOR COLLAGEN

When you eat a collagen-rich food, your body (specifically your digestive enzymes) breaks that collagen down into its individual amino acids and peptide parts. It takes a bit of time and effort, and it's unclear how much of the collagen and beneficial molecules actually make it into your body. But animal-sourced collagen is the most natural form of supplementing your own collagen supply, getting more essential amino acids, and helping your body produce more of the helpful protein.

WHY SUPPLEMENTS ARE GOOD FOR COLLAGEN

With hydrolyzed collagen, the work of breaking down the collagen has already been done for you. *Hydrolyzed* means heated, and when collagen is heated, the molecules shrink as the helices unwind. The collagen chains also break into smaller pieces. That lets your intestines and stomach get to the work of absorbing the amino acids and peptides quickly, so ultimately they may be absorbed more efficiently than collagen found in foods. However, this is not yet confirmed, as researchers are still trying to understand how well the body handles collagen from both sources.

HOW DO COLLAGEN SUPPLEMENTS WORK?

If your body begins to make less collagen with age, can you replace it with a supplement? Not exactly, but collagen supplements might be highly beneficial and can ultimately increase your collagen levels. Here's how.

Collagen supplements are animal-derived products. Collagen from animal products, like fish and pork skin, is processed until it's broken down into a powdery supplement. When you take that supplement, either as a powder in food or as a pill, you end up providing your body with a dose of amino acids, vitamins, minerals, and collagen molecules. Your body can then take those

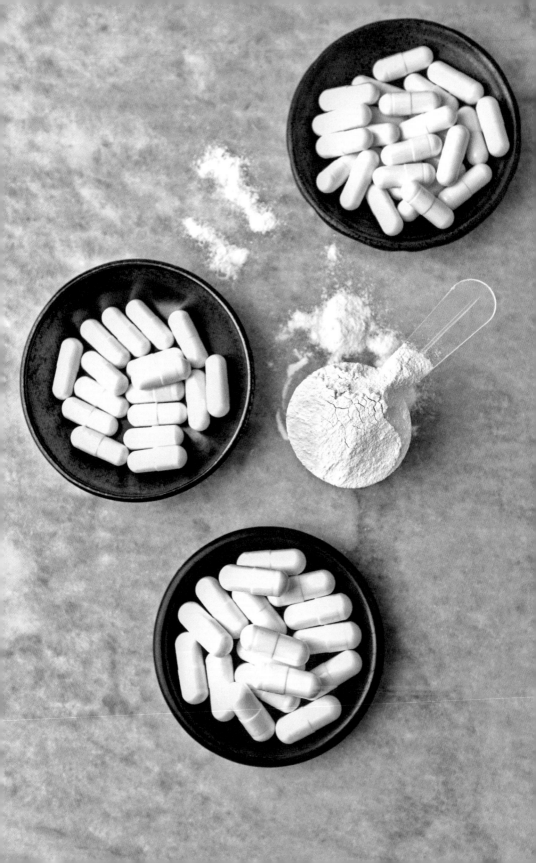

elements and deliver them throughout your systems, or in the case of the amino acids, it'll use those elements to form new collagen.

WHAT'S BETTER: FOOD OR SUPPLEMENT?

Both food and supplements are good, though it will likely be easier to get collagen from supplements because food sources are so limited. You should still look to help your body produce more of its own proteins—by eating collagen-boosting foods, for example—and you can look to supplement your daily diet with peptides. It's not always easy to eat as well as you should, whether it's for the purposes of increasing collagen or just in general, so a supplement might be helpful.

HOW CAN YOU KNOW COLLAGEN IS GOING WHERE YOU WANT IT?

To put it simply, you can't. When you eat collagen from food or take a collagen supplement, you're increasing your supply of the amino acids and molecules that are needed to build collagen, promote collagen development, and replace lost collagen. You can't, for example, take a supplement only for the purposes of boosting elasticity in your skin.

The expression "a rising tide lifts all boats" comes to mind when thinking about how collagen works in the body. Eating collagen or supplementing with a collagen powder increases your overall collagen levels and your ability to manufacture the protein naturally. You can be taking it because you want to see younger, more supple skin, but the benefits may show up in many places simply because collagen accumulates where it wants.

Types I and III collagen have specific benefits—for the skin, for example— whereas type II is best for cartilage. This is about as specific as you can get with selecting the benefit you want from the collagen supplements or collagen foods you eat currently. More research may tell us additional information.

GELATIN VS. COLLAGEN

Often, gelatin and collagen are used interchangeably, and while they are very closely related—gelatin does come from collagen—they're different enough that you should know how to talk about them as separate elements.

Perhaps the easiest way to consider how gelatin and collagen connect is to think of bone broth. Bones (or skin, shells, or other connective tissues) are placed in a large vat of water and slowly cooked over the course of a day or two. During this slow process, the bones leak their collagen into the broth and the collagen begins to break down.

The gelatin that forms can then be taken and processed even further to form hydrolyzed collagen, or the powdery supplement sold as collagen peptides.

Gelatin, on the other hand, is dried and then turned into sheets or granules. In order to use gelatin in food, you'll first have to "bloom" it by placing the gelatin sheets or capsules in water and letting them plump up. Then you can take the hydrated protein and add it to a hot liquid so it can fully break down and be absorbed into the food.

Both gelatin and collagen have about 10 grams of collagen per tablespoon (or 20 grams for a two-tablespoon scoop, which is commonly included in supplement jars). Which you decide to use largely depends on how much time you have and what you want to use it for. Gelatin often retains a meaty flavor. It's rarely processed enough to remove the flavor components of the animal elements from which it was rendered. Collagen peptides, on the other hand, can be purchased as a flavorless product or one that's been flavored with other ingredients, like chocolate or vanilla.

There is one benefit to gelatin that collagen does not offer. Gelatin "sticks" around in your gastrointestinal system a bit longer. Because it's not as highly processed as hydrolyzed collagen, gelatin is slower to break down once consumed. Gelatin also coats the intestines as it travels from top to bottom in the gastrointestinal (GI) tract. That may be beneficial for people with some GI health issues, including leaky gut or irritable bowel syndromes.

* **The basic difference:** When collagen breaks down, it becomes gelatin

Fast Facts

Supplements might be the easiest and most effective way to boost your collagen supply and encourage your tissues to make more of their own collagen, but foods that already have collagen happen to be delicious. There's no harm in eating collagen-rich foods *and* taking collagen supplements. Even in large doses, collagen has shown no harmful side effects.

EVERYTHING YOU NEED TO KNOW ABOUT COLLAGEN POWDER

You can, and certainly should, try to eat collagen-rich foods if and when you can, but you'll likely need to supplement natural collagen sources because collagen from animal products is either difficult to get (bone marrow) or takes a great deal of time and effort to prepare (bone broth).

HOW ARE COLLAGEN POWDERS MADE?

Collagen is extracted from the richest sources of protein: eggshells, cattle and pig bones, fish scales, animal tissues, etc. The process typically involves a long, slow heating process (akin to making bone broth) that allows the protein gelatin to be extracted from the collagen. That gelatin is further processed to break down some of its elements and make the supplement easier to absorb. What's left is a fine, chalky powder that you may recognize in the large plastic tubs that are sold in vitamin stores and grocery stores today.

Bovine (Beef or Cow) Collagen

Bovine collagen is sourced primarily from the skin, bones, and muscles of cattle. This type of collagen is abundant in collagen types I and III, and it's a good source of glycine and proline. Bovine collagen is especially helpful for boosting collagen production and helping the body build muscle mass.

Chicken Collagen

Chicken stands alone as one of the best sources of type II collagen. This type is especially great for supporting cartilage and connective tissues. It's also a good source of glucosamine sulfate and chondroitin sulfate, natural compounds that are linked to better joint health.

Marine (Fish) Collagen

Marine, or piscine, collagen comes from the bones and skin of fish. Type I collagen is most prominent in these animal parts, as are the amino acids glycine, proline, and hydroxyproline. Research suggests marine collagen may be most beneficial for joint health, cardiovascular health, and digestive health.

Egg Collagen

Egg collagen is found in the white, yolk, and shell membrane. (You don't have to eat the shells, but they're good if you're ever making chicken bone broth.) Eggs are richest in types I, III, and V, but they have one hundred times more type I collagen than their second-most abundant type of collagen (V). Egg collagen is also a good source of glycine, proline, and hydroxyproline, as it's host to eighteen total amino acids.

HOW IS HYDROLYZED COLLAGEN MADE?

To hydrolyze collagen, manufacturers heat it. Heating helps the collagen helices unwind, and the molecules begin to shrink. Collagen molecules from many food sources are simply too large for your body to absorb—though that's not a reason not to eat them when you can. Shrinking them increases the percentage of collagen molecules that will make it past your gastrointestinal system and to your joints, ligaments, skin, bones, or wherever else the protein is needed.

WHERE DO I USE COLLAGEN POWDER?

Collagen powder manufacturers suggest using protein powders in any place you'd normally use protein powders, from smoothies and soups to drinks and even ice pops. Collagen peptides can be used hot or cold, whereas gelatin needs to be heated to thoroughly dissolve.

You can go simple with your collagen supplementation: stir it into a morning cup of coffee or even a glass of water. Or you can be as complicated and involved as you want.

If you don't want to use a powder, your other option (bone broth) is a little more labor-intensive and can take several days depending on your method. But at the end of it, you have the equivalent of collagen liquid gold.

CAN I BUY A VEGAN COLLAGEN POWDER?

No. If you see a product labeled as a vegan collagen powder, you're looking at a fake. Collagen cannot be a plant-based product because plants don't contain collagen; only animal proteins, specifically connective tissue and bones, have the protein.

If you see a product promoting itself as a source of vegan collagen, what you're actually looking at is a supplement with amino acids, vitamins, and minerals. Sure, some of those elements may help make collagen molecules and fibrils down the line, but they aren't collagen.

A WORD ABOUT SOURCING

The quality of the collagen you get from animal protein is only as good as the quality of the product you buy. Many conventionally raised animals won't have high-quality collagen in their bones, hide, or joints because they're not raised in such a way as to encourage this type of growth. (They're fed to make more beef.)

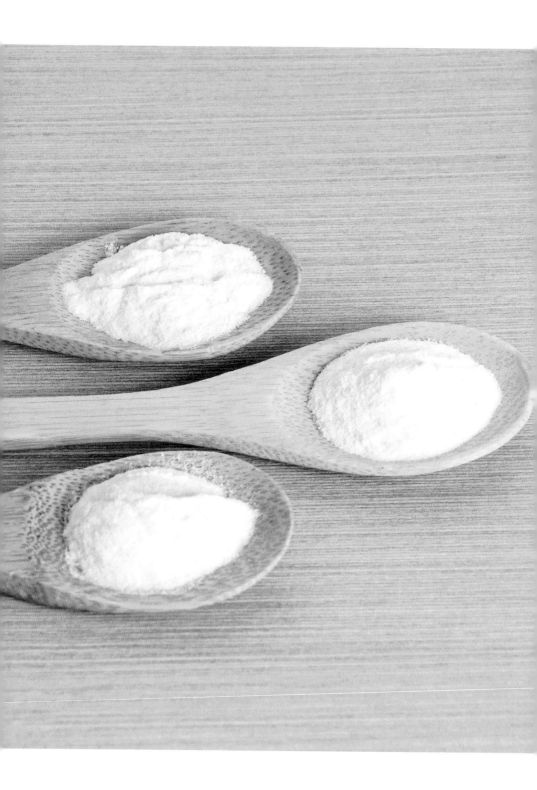

COLLAGEN HANDBOOK

When you're buying, ideally your sources of collagen will come from grass-fed, pasture-raised beef that is not treated with antibiotics or hormones to grow larger faster. Research brands before buying. Ones that spend the effort (and, honestly, the money) to make their collagen in this sustainable, healthy fashion are often more expensive. But in the end, you have a better product that's delivering healthier proteins, and you are supporting a less cruel, non-factory-farmed process.

WHAT TO LOOK FOR IN A COLLAGEN POWDER

When you're at the store or shopping online, keep these factors in mind as you pick a product that you intend to use.

Buy Hydrolyzed Collagen

This type of collagen has been processed to a point that it's more easily absorbed by your body—specifically your intestines. The smaller collagen molecules in hydrolyzed collagen can more quickly and efficiently move from your digestive system to other portions of your body.

Look for Vitamin C

Some companies, knowing how vital vitamin C is to the collagen synthesis process, add a vitamin C supplement to the collagen product. Read the labels, and if your preferred product doesn't have any vitamin C or ascorbic acid, consider taking a supplement or increasing your intake of vitamin C–rich foods in order to reap the most collagen-production reward from the supplement you're taking.

Consider Sweeteners, Artificial Flavors, and Preservatives

Collagen supplements have come a long way from their mysterious chalky powder state of earlier years. Today's collagen companies manufacture products that have unique flavors like berry, vanilla, and even matcha. Some of the supplements, unfortunately, use artificial flavorings and sweeteners to pique consumer interest and possibly make the mystifying product less perplexing. (Admirable, but not necessary.)

Before you buy, consider what's right for you. Artificial sweeteners, for example, can cause gastric distress and headaches in the short-term. Some people may have allergic reactions to them; they can even increase inflammation.

The American Heart Association and American Diabetes Association® have given a reluctant nod to artificial sweeteners in place of full-calorie sweeteners. Of course, the goal of their approval is to encourage the use of these alternative sweeteners as a means to combat America's worsening obesity epidemic. If you prefer sweeter applications for collagen supplements, consider what type of sweetener is right for your lifestyle and your dietary strategy.

WHERE DO I BUY COLLAGEN POWDER?

You can find collagen supplements at any number of grocery stores, health food chains, vitamin stores, and online retailers. See page 145 for a list of recommended brands.

HOW MUCH COLLAGEN SHOULD I TAKE?

No recommended daily value exists for collagen, as it's still new. It's also not considered a necessary or vital supplement, so setting a standard largely relies on looking at amounts used in studies and drawing conclusions based on reactions and any adverse effects that occurred, if any.

With that in mind, the average person can take between 2.5 and 12 grams of a collagen supplement each day and reap the rewards. The majority of studies that have looked at the potential benefits of collagen have used amounts in that range. Some have used more, even as much as 15 grams, but no additional benefit for the higher amount was found.

Future studies may be able to determine more precise dosing recommendations. For now, you can begin with smaller doses—2.5 grams, for example—and if you experience no side effects, you can begin slowly increasing until you reach a point that feels right for you. You can also consult your doctor or a registered dietitian who may be able to help you decide on a dose that is reasonable and likely to provide the benefits you're seeking.

ARE THERE SIDE EFFECTS OR RISKS?

Few side effects are reported with the use of collagen. Those that do occur are typically related to the gastrointestinal system. They include upset stomach, nausea, and bloating. These reactions are more common in people who take a too-large dose or have an allergy.

If you have a food allergy, you'll want to steer clear of collagen supplements that use collagen processed from the source of your allergic reaction. You can read the label to determine if the food to which you're allergic is present. If the product lists collagen types only, this guide will come in handy:

COLLAGEN SOURCES BY TYPE
In most cases, these collagen types are
sourced from the following proteins.

Type I: bovine, fish, and eggs

Type II: chicken

Type III: bovine, fish, and eggs

Type V: eggs

IS COLLAGEN RIGHT FOR ME?

Before you load up on plastic tubs of collagen and whip up your first collagen-fortified green smoothie, it's important to place what we know about collagen in a larger context.

For the past few decades, doctors have suspected that the role collagen plays in our health, well-being, and physical development is far greater than first understood. Indeed, the scope of collagen's responsibilities is vast, and each new study sheds more light on the important role it plays.

But collagen research is still relatively new—and by that I mean there isn't a great deal of information out there for doctors, dietitians, and other nutrition experts to use as a firm foundation on which to make recommendations.

That means the choice is yours. The good news is that collagen research has found negative effects rare and mostly mild when they do occur. In dozens of studies, moderately high doses of collagen, around 10 grams, have been shown to produce helpful benefits and noticeable, even measurable, results. If you think collagen sounds like a good fit for your lifestyle, you can certainly try it. Give it a few months; most reports suggest that true benefits take up to six months to become quantifiable. If you feel a difference, or if blood results suggest there's been an improvement over that timeframe, you may be seeing a concrete example of how the protein can help people.

IMPORTANT NOTE: If you're thinking of using a supplement to treat a collagen-related condition or disease, such as brittle bone disease or osteoarthritis, don't turn your back on traditional methods entirely without first consulting a doctor. While research does show promising signs, especially as it relates to osteoarthritis and bone and joint health, it's nowhere near conclusive enough to reject the traditional methods that, in many cases, have been found to be beneficial.

If you have a collagen-related condition or one you think might be improved by the use of collagen supplements, talk with your doctor. The two of you can weigh the benefits with the risks. The choice to supplement with a collagen powder shouldn't be made without first considering the other treatments you're already taking.

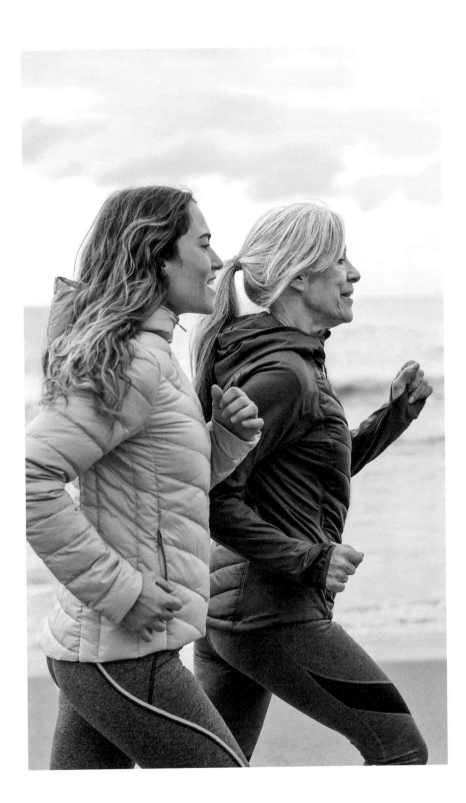

All About Collagen

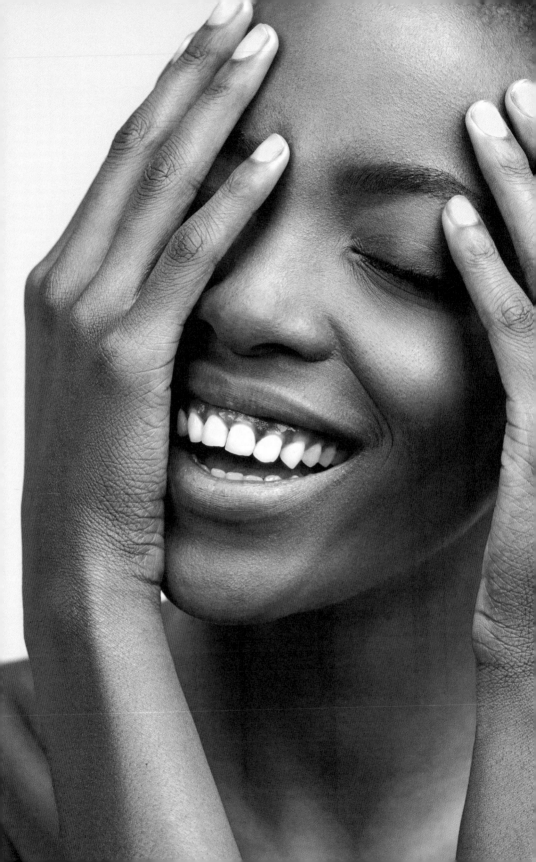

PART 2

Skin Health

I n your skin, collagen is both the structure—it binds together the many cells and layers of skin to form the largest organ we have—and the "filling." Where collagen cells are present in abundance, a rich network of collagen makes skin appear supple and full.

When collagen cells are depleted, the skin becomes thin and less flexible. Signs of aging become more obvious, too, as skin sags, wrinkles develop, and lines deepen.

COLLAGEN: THE FOUNTAIN OF YOUTH?

How you age is one part genetic and one part environmental. Your DNA, your lifestyle, and your skin-protective choices may play the role of judge and jury for your skin's appearance as you grow older.

At the same time, the collagen content of your skin's surfaces decreases approximately 1 percent per year. Decelerating or even supplementing this collagen loss may be the key to slowing visible aging.

It's no wonder, then, that collagen is one of the leading areas of research for reversing the signs of aging. Collagen could be a superhero of sorts, one that sweeps in to save your day—or rather, to save your skin.

Reduces Signs of Aging

The market for nutricosmetic products—dietary supplements you take for potential benefits like enhancing skin hydration or reducing signs of aging—is hot and shows little sign of cooling. However, research is limited, and it's unclear how great the impact of these products can be. Many of the beneficial components in these pills, capsules, or powders are often broken down and destroyed by acids and enzymes in the digestive tract before they can be absorbed and transported through the body.

With collagen, that does not appear to be the case. In fact, research has shown that hydrolyzed collagen can be absorbed by the intestines and will produce observable, measurable changes. Some, in fact, are noticeable in as little as four weeks.

Promotes Elasticity

Collagen forms an immense network in the top two layers of your skin—the epidermis and dermis. As you age, this network begins to fragment, which can lead to less flexibility and elasticity.

One study found that people who took 2.5 to 5 grams of collagen supplements every day for eight weeks saw statistically significant improvement over the placebo participants. These skin benefits remained at a four-week follow-up after the end of the study, even when participants were no longer taking the collagen supplement.

Increases Skin Moisture

Decreased skin hydration is an early and long-lasting sign of aging. Boosting hydration can help improve signs of aging as well as other appearance-related skin issues. Oral collagen supplements show great promise in reversing this element of skin aging.

One eight-week study found that taking collagen peptide supplements led to significantly increased skin hydration. The density of collagen in the skin was also significantly bolstered, and collagen fragmentation, or the breakdown of the collagen network that occurs with aging, decreased. In fact, the study showed that fragmentation had slowed in as little as four weeks.

Reduces Wrinkle Depth

As your skin's network of collagen strands and cells begins to fragment and break apart, fine lines and wrinkles will develop. You may notice them first around your eyes, mouth, or nose, but the loss of collagen is also responsible for visible lines and wrinkles on your hands, chest, and neck.

But one study found that a nutritional supplement beverage containing collagen peptides as well as a mixture of vitamins, minerals, and hyaluronic acid, significantly reduced the depth of facial wrinkles. It also improved skin hydration and elasticity, which can further decrease the appearance of lines and wrinkles.

Diminishes Cellulite

In addition to fine lines and wrinkles, cellulite is a common skin problem about which many people complain, but one study suggests that taking a collagen supplement may also improve signs of that age-related skin condition.

In the study, 105 normal-weight and overweight women were given either 2.5 grams of collagen peptides or a placebo every day for six months. The signs and severity of their collagen were assessed at the beginning of the study and then again three and six months later, when the study had concluded. In women of normal weight, taking collagen resulted in a significant decrease in the degree of cellulite. It also reduced visible skin waviness on the thighs.

Overweight women had some improvement, but not any that came to a level of statistical significance. Still, for women concerned about cellulite, a collagen supplement may be one way to help erase some of the visible signs.

SKIN CARE THAT SHOWS: ANTIOXIDANTS CAN BOOST COLLAGEN

Vitamins, antioxidants, and polyphenols are esteemed for their many healthful benefits, including reducing the risk of many diseases. For your skin, these nutrients can also help reduce signs of aging by slowing how rapidly collagen breaks down. They may also eliminate free radicals, the molecules associated with increased risk of disease.

Getting adequate amounts of these vitamins and minerals in your daily diet can not only boost your overall health, but also increase collagen production, which can have an antiaging effect.

Vitamin C

One study found that vitamin C supplements can boost the production of type I and type III collagens. Vitamin C also induces the production of enzymes that encourage your body's own natural collagen development. Without vitamin C, your body cannot convert amino acids into the strands that form collagen fibrils.

Vitamin E

Taking vitamin C with vitamin E may have a doubly profound impact on skin health. Research shows that the benefit of these two antioxidants together is more impactful than either of the vitamins alone.

TOPICAL COLLAGEN FOR SKIN

If consuming collagen through food or supplements has a beneficial impact on skin health and appearance, it stands to reason that applying topical collagen-boosting products or nutrients might also have a beneficial impact. And you'd be correct.

While the primary focus of this book is on foods and oral supplements for improving collagen network development and increasing circulating collagen in your body's cells, it's important to know collagen has benefits as a topical application as well.

Cosmetics that promote peptides or collagen as an ingredient, including lotions, ointments, and creams, may have a beneficial impact on your skin's appearance. As they do inside the body, many of these products not only supplement the collagen you have in your skin, they can also induce your body's own natural collagen production.

Vitamin A

Retinol (vitamin A) is a type of antioxidant, and like vitamin C and E supplements, research suggests it can have a strong impact on the body's natural collagen metabolism and can speed up cell turnover. These two actions can lead to smoother skin, reduced fine lines, and an overall improved appearance.

Peptides

Collagen peptides can be added to topical treatments. In the body, peptides can even imitate the molecules of collagen, potentially causing the body to make more of its own collagen.

BID BRITTLE NAILS ADIEU

Thin, brittle nails don't just make for a lackluster manicure; thin nails can break and snag and may cause painful tears or bleeding. Collagen, however, may help fortify your nails to grow stronger and longer without chips, cracks, or breaks.

In one study, twenty-five participants were given 2.5 grams of collagen peptides every day for twenty-four weeks. At the end of the study period, the participants reported significant changes:

* 12 percent saw increased nail growth

* 42 percent experienced fewer broken nails

* 64 percent reported seeing an overall improvement to their formerly brittle nails

And even more surprisingly, almost nine in ten participants (88 percent) said the changes were noticeable by week four.

Fast Facts

Your body continually makes collagen throughout your life, but as you age, it makes less and less. This invites signs of aging, like loss of skin hydration and increased fine lines and deep wrinkles. Research suggests that collagen supplementation can help slow these signs of aging. Consuming collagen, whether in supplement or food form, may help ease dryness, reduce wrinkle depth, improve skin structure, and boost elasticity.

HEALTHIER JOINTS

Articular cartilage is the rubbery, smooth connective tissue that covers the ends of bones where they come together to form your joints. Think of cartilage as a cushion that protects bones during movement. When you use your joints in everyday motion, they absorb a lot of weight and impact. Cartilage helps prevent pain or discomfort and keeps bones protected with all of those movements.

Cartilage also allows for easier joint rotation. It acts as a natural gliding pad so your joints can move more smoothly, without the risk of painful friction.

Collagen is the primary component of cartilage. Both the extracellular matrix (ECM) and two-thirds of the body's cartilage mass are created from various types of collagen. Cartilage is strong and supple in your early years, but wear and tear, age, and collagen deterioration all have an impact. Over time, the cartilage can turn thin, become inflexible, or disappear entirely.

As cartilage becomes thinner, it becomes less effective, leaving little cushioning in your joints and increasing your risk for degenerative joint disorders, such as osteoarthritis (OA). This type of joint deterioration can lead to painful symptoms like cracking or clicking when you move the affected joint and swelling and inflammation, as well as a limited range of motion. OA occurs most often in large joints like knees, hips, and the lower back, but it can also affect the neck, fingers, and toes.

One in two adults in the United States will develop OA of the knee in their lifetime. One in four will have some form of the degenerative arthritis by the time they're eighty-five years old. As such, it's one of the leading causes of chronic disability in the United States.

There is no cure for OA, and conventional treatments are limited in their ability to provide real, lasting relief. Pain medication provides some mild relief, especially for inflammation and swelling, but long-term use may be problematic. Corticosteroids can also reduce inflammation, but frequent use carries risks, such as high blood pressure, fluid retention, and elevated pressure in the eyes. Ultimately, joint replacement is considered, to repair or replace the affected joint entirely.

Because of the problematic nature of many OA treatments, researchers and doctors have long considered alternative treatments that might help slow the progression of OA or prevent it entirely. Collagen is one such area of interest.

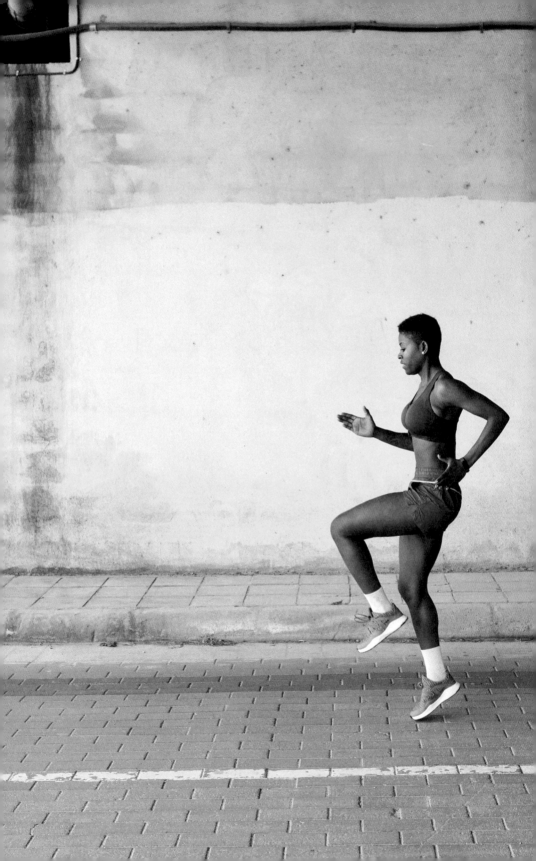

COLLAGEN: THE ULTIMATE PAIN RELIEVER?

Research suggests collagen might have two important roles to play in making joints healthier and stronger. One study found that once collagen is absorbed in the intestines, it then accumulates preferentially in cartilage and bones. That means you can boost your own natural stores of collagen by taking supplements.

Secondarily, additional studies have shown that taking collagen supplements may stimulate your body's own natural collagen production. This could lead to a boost in the extracellular matrix of cartilage and may help slow the natural deterioration of the all-important joint coverings. This can have several important benefits for your joints.

Bolsters Cartilage

With age and activity, cartilage begins to wear away. That means the extracellular matrix and web of collagen cells that make up cartilage also begin to deteriorate.

One conventional OA treatment that aims to retain collagen in cartilage is hyaluronic acid injections. This substance is found naturally in your skin and connective tissues. It acts to keep your tissues lubricated for easier movement and reduced friction. Hyaluronic acid also helps cartilage retain its natural collagen. Injections, in that way, can help to both increase joint mobility and prevent additional collagen loss.

Taken along or in combination with hyaluronic acid injections, collagen supplements may be one way to naturally boost the collagen in your cartilage. Research shows collagen supplements not only provide additional cartilage to your body's tissues and organs but can also stimulate production of the protein. Taking steps to maintain the collagen you have while also adding to it could be beneficial to joints that have suffered cartilage loss.

Prevents Joint Deterioration

Supplementing natural collagen and bolstering it with collagen peptides may prevent the loss of cartilage. Sustaining a protective layer of cartilage around bones and in joints can have long-term benefits. Once the cartilage is gone, bones begin to rub against each other. This can lead to painful symptoms and disability.

Provides Pain Relief

Over-the-counter pain medications are commonly recommended to individuals with mild to moderate joint pain and even to those with diagnosed OA. But research suggests you may be able to put down your bottle of pills if you begin taking collagen supplements.

You don't even need chronic joint pain to benefit from collagen supplements. Even acute pain—that is, temporary joint pain perhaps caused by overexertion or a minor injury—may be reduced in people with regular collagen intake. In a twenty-four-week study of seventy-three college athletes, participants who took collagen hydrolysate (a product of collagen hydrolysis) experienced less joint pain at rest, when walking, when standing, when carrying objects, and when lifting. They also had significantly less knee pain.

This study bolsters the idea that taking collagen before you have any joint deterioration or are experiencing other issues may have some protective benefits. Indeed, as the authors of this study concluded, this may point to the idea that taking supplemental collagen could reduce your risk of joint deterioration, especially if you already have an increased risk.

Eases Osteoarthritis Symptoms

With stronger, more fortified cartilage and joints that are increasingly protected against tissue deterioration, it stands to reason that people with osteoarthritis who are taking collagen may experience fewer symptoms of the degenerative joint disease. Indeed, one study of eighty individuals with OA of the hip or knee found this to be the case. In a seventy-day study, participants were given a collagen product made with chicken cartilage. During the study, the participants met with researchers who measured their pain and OA symptoms on multiple scales.

By one scale, patients reported a reduction in pain in as little as thirty-five days. By day seventy, both scales showed significant improvement in the physical symptoms of osteoarthritis. Some of the study participants were even able to engage in physical activities they had avoided previously because of OA symptoms.

What Are the Symptoms of Osteoarthritis?

Osteoarthritis (OA) is the degeneration of joint cartilage and, eventually, bone. For most people, early symptoms begin in middle age, but overexertion or frequent use of any joint can lead to damage and, in time, cartilage breakdown.

The most common symptoms of OA include:

* pain
* stiffness, particularly in the morning or after periods of rest
* swelling after prolonged use
* limited range of motion

As OA worsens and more cartilage wears away, you may experience painful bone-on-bone contact. This may cause:

* cracking or clicking sounds when using the joint
* chronic inflammation around the joint
* a grating or scraping sensation when moving the joint

Over time, OA may make everyday activities more difficult and increasingly painful. Simple tasks, like holding a coffee cup or grasping a pen to write, may become nearly impossible.

If joints in your lower body, such as the hips or knees, are affected, then walking, sitting, standing, or climbing stairs may be difficult. Loss of joint mobility may make you unstable on your feet and more likely to fall.

Fast Facts

Collagen is a primary component of cartilage, the rubbery, protective tissue that surrounds the ends of bones and makes joints move smoothly. When cartilage begins to thin and disappear, painful symptoms can set in. But research suggests bolstering collagen content in your cartilage may slow tissue loss and ease symptoms. Collagen supplementation may also help your tissues make more of their own natural cartilage. This can lead to reduced inflammation and pain relief. It may also ward off joint disorders like osteoarthritis.

GOOD FOR THE HEART

Just as collagen provides structure and support to muscles all over the body, it also comprises the body's arteries and blood vessels. Collagen keeps these vital portions of your cardiovascular system nimble but strong. Without collagen, the arteries could weaken and reach a potentially dangerous fragile state.

This could increase the risk for atherosclerosis, a disease that causes narrowing in your arteries. Over time, this can lead to potentially dangerous and deadly complications, including heart attack and stroke.

Few studies have looked at the impact collagen might have on the heart, blood vessels, arteries, and overall cardiovascular system, but the ones that have show some promise.

COLLAGEN: THE HEART HEALER?

As previously explained, collagen is composed of several amino acids—glycine, proline, arginine, and hydroxyproline. In addition to forming collagen, however, these amino acids have several other significant functions, from repairing wounds (arginine) to promoting sleep (glycine). Research also suggests they may work together to provide significant cardiovascular benefits as well.

Reduces Artery Stiffness

Artery stiffness is a key risk factor for cardiovascular disease. Stiff arteries are less able to transport blood smoothly, and clots can form within the narrowed, hardened walls, which could lead to stroke or heart attack. In one study of thirty-one adults, researchers gave the participants 16 grams of a collagen supplement every day for the six-month study. At the end, participants showed significant reductions in measures that detect artery stiffness.

Boosts HDL, Lowers LDL

In that same study, the thirty-one participants also saw their high-density lipoprotein (HDL)—the good kind of cholesterol—rise by an average of

6 percent. Healthy levels of HDL—and low levels of its counterpart, low-density lipoprotein (LDL)—can decrease the risk for heart disease and heart conditions like atherosclerosis.

Another study saw similar blood cholesterol changes. In this study, fifty participants took marine collagen peptides, or collagen derived from fish, for three months. At the end of the study period, blood tests showed a significant drop in LDL levels as well as an increase in HDL.

Decreases Blood Pressure

In addition to the changes in blood cholesterol, the study participants who took marine collagen also saw a drop in their diastolic blood pressure (the reading at the bottom of a blood pressure measurement) and their arterial pressure. Both of these significant results point to better heart health and a decreased risk of hypertension and other heart-related conditions.

Fast Facts

More research is needed to understand the impact collagen can have on creating a healthier cardiovascular system and reducing the risk for heart-related conditions like atherosclerosis. However, existing studies point to several significant possible benefits as well as the need to continue studying the use of this protein in treating heart-related issues.

BETTER BONES

Collagen is the primary protein found in bones. It forms a soft framework that gives each bone its structure. The mineral calcium phosphate adds strength and hardens the bones so they can withstand force and movement.

Bones are constantly reinforcing themselves. As older minerals and collagen cells disintegrate, newer ones replace them so your bones stay strong and support your muscles and limbs. However, bone loss eventually outpaces bone replacement.

Throughout the earliest years of life, bone creation happens more quickly than bone matter loss. It's in these prime years that we build and store the bone mineral density that will sustain us throughout our lives. Peak bone density occurs in the late twenties. By age thirty, you will have as much bone density as you're ever going to have.

From that point on, bones slowly lose their density. Bone loss accelerates in women in the first few years after menopause.

If your bones lose too much mass or become porous, you may develop a condition called osteoporosis. More than fifty million Americans experience osteoporosis. This condition increases your risk of bone fractures, joint pain, and reduced mobility.

WHAT ARE THE SYMPTOMS OF OSTEOPOROSIS?

Osteoporosis is a condition that causes bones to become porous, brittle, and weak. As bones become more fragile, they're more likely to fracture or break. This can lead to long-term disability, painful surgery, and, in some cases, even death.

Osteoporosis is an underdiagnosed and undertreated condition. That's because osteoporosis is considered a silent disease; many individuals do not realize they have bone deterioration until they experience a fall or an accident that results in a broken or dislocated bone.

X-rays or other imaging scans will reveal the result of porous bones as well as the extent of deterioration. Bone density tests are available, and they're recommended for women over age sixty-five and for those with multiple risk factors.

COLLAGEN: THE BONE BUILDER?

Research suggests supplemental collagen may improve bone density and preserve bone health. In menopausal women, it may also slow collagen loss.

Though you cannot stop the slow deterioration of bone mass, you may be able to add to your collagen stores with supplements. Increasing the amount of collagen available to your bones could help prevent serious complications associated with weak bones and bone density loss.

Reduces Collagen Breakdown

A great deal of bone loss is tied to collagen loss, which also increases with age. Without a vast collagen framework, bones have less structure and less strength. Therefore, it stands to reason that adding more collagen to your body may slow collagen (and bone) loss.

Indeed, one study found that taking a collagen hydrolysate with the added hormone calcitonin may reduce collagen breakdown. In the study, more than one hundred postmenopausal women with osteoporosis were given a treatment with both collagen and calcitonin. At the end of the twenty-four-week study period, the participants had marginal improvements in bone mass loss, but they showed a significant reduction in the markers that signal collagen is breaking down. If you can prevent collagen loss, you may be able to prevent bone loss.

Sustains Bone Strength

Bones can deteriorate with age due to wear and tear as well as loss of bone density. Collagen may help bones maintain their strength, and it may encourage collagen proliferation in bones and surrounding joint structures.

In one study focusing on rats, researchers found that the group that received the highest dose of collagen hydrolysate withstood four times as heavy a weight as rats that received a smaller dose. They also had higher bone protein and mineral content. Additional research in humans is needed to replicate the same results, but small-scale studies have shown benefits to bone strength in people taking supplemental collagen.

Boosts Bone Mineral Density

With age, all-important minerals may leach from bones. Research suggests, however, that hydrolyzed collagen supplements can increase bone mineral density (BMD), which is a measure of the amount of minerals, such as calcium, in your bones. Low BMD is tied to fragile bones and osteoporosis.

In a study of 102 postmenopausal women with age-related BMD loss, researchers discovered that 5 grams of collagen peptides increased BMD during the course of the twelve-month study. The women who took the collagen saw a 7 percent increase on average in their BMD compared to women who took a placebo.

Slows Bone Mineral Density Loss

Calcium, a mineral that also helps build bone strength, may be beneficial when taken with a collagen supplement. In one study of thirty-nine women, those who took a combination of 5 grams of collagen, calcium, and vitamin D saw substantially lower BMD loss than women who took the calcium and vitamin D without collagen.

By the end of the twelve-month study, the women who took the collagen supplement combination also had significantly lower levels of proteins that promote bone breakdown and BMD loss in their blood. That portends a longer-lasting protective effect that could keep bones from losing minerals as quickly as they might naturally.

Fast Facts

Though limited, research in humans suggests that taking supplemental collagen may help slow bone collagen loss, preserve bone mineral density, and reduce mineral loss and bone breakdown. This can lead to improved mobility, and it can reduce your risk of osteoporosis and similar bone conditions.

BUILD STRONGER MUSCLES

Muscles, like bones, are made from a combination of substances. In the case of bones, it's collagen and minerals. In the case of muscles, the collection includes connective tissues, nerves, blood vessels, contractile tissue—and, yes, collagen.

Like bones, muscle mass begins to deteriorate with age. Even the most devoted weight lifters experience strength reduction as muscle tissue diminishes and the percentage of muscle to other tissue shrinks.

Unlike bones, however, there is an element of maintenance or muscle building you can do. Resistance training and weight lifting help stimulate muscle tissue growth. Protein supplements like collagen may boost that process, too.

COLLAGEN: JUST LIKE LIFTING WEIGHTS?

While collagen accounts for only 1 to 10 percent of muscle tissue, research suggests protein can play a significant role in boosting muscle mass and possibly even stimulating muscle growth. You may just need to take collagen *and* lift weights to see the most benefit.

Increases Muscle Mass

Some skeletal muscle tissue loss is natural. With age, tissue grows weaker and muscle strands are less forceful. This process is called sarcopenia, and studies suggest that people with sarcopenia may actually be able to recover some muscle mass with collagen supplements.

In fact, in one study of fifty-three men with sarcopenia, half were given a 15-gram protein supplement that contained collagen. At the same time, they took part in a twelve-week guided resistance-training program with lessons three times per week. At the end of the study, the twenty-seven men who took the collagen supplements *and* did the resistance training had greater muscle mass and less fat mass in their bodies.

Increases Muscle Strength

In that same study of older men with sarcopenia, researchers discovered that the twelve-week resistance-training program combined with collagen peptide supplements boosted muscle strength. The control group, which did the resistance training but did not take the collagen supplement, saw some increased muscle strength at the end of the program, but the impact was more significant in the combination-treatment group.

May Stimulate Muscle Growth

Researchers hypothesize that taking dietary proteins (collagen) when in a muscle-training program may increase muscle synthesis and decrease muscle breakdown. In particular, studies suggest that the addition of a collagen supplement to a resistance-training program could boost the body's own production of creatine and muscle proteins. This may stimulate muscle growth and help one rebound from age-related muscle loss.

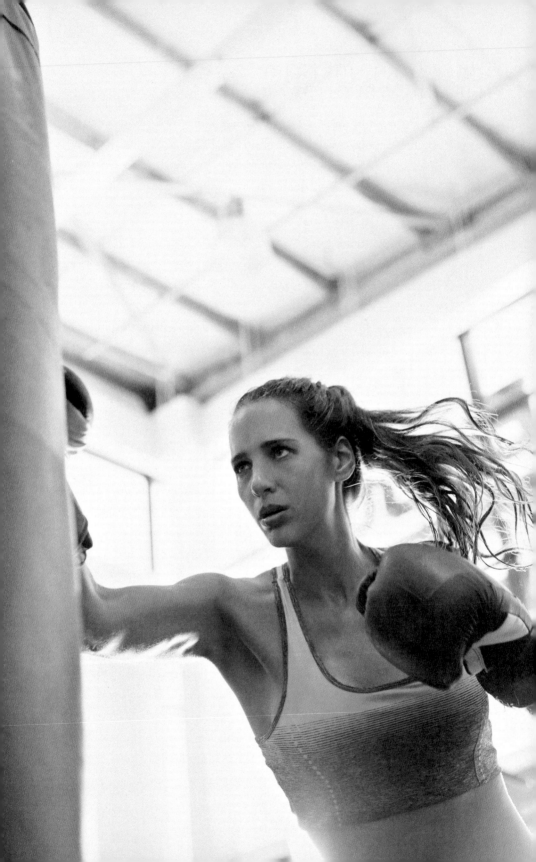

Fast Facts

Collagen supplements may boost muscle growth or slow down age-related muscle deterioration. Taking collagen with a resistance-training regimen may also help individuals increase strength, even if they do not currently have any muscle mass loss.

OTHER POSSIBLE BENEFITS

Collagen is still a relatively new area of research for scientists. Though it's been recognized as an important protein and essential to so many parts of the body, from eyes to nails, it's only been in the last two decades that dedicated research has shifted focus to its many possible benefits.

That means some areas of benefit are well known—strengthening joints, building stronger joints, and improving signs of aging, for example—and some are just now burgeoning and garnering attention, whether through anecdotal evidence or small studies with promising results that merit larger, more intense investigations.

Keep in mind that these benefits are supported by a handful of studies or just a bit of research. It's not enough to bank on, but it's something to watch for the future.

May Prevent Dementia

Your brain is formed in large part by collagen-rich structures, from cartilage and muscle down to the neurons that send signals throughout your body. In one study, researchers discovered that type IV collagen may have protective benefits against the plaque buildup of Alzheimer's disease.

In the study, researchers found that this particular type of collagen prevents amyloid-beta plaques from developing and attacking neurons. Amyloid-beta is a type of amino acid. It's "sticky" and clumps together to form the devastating plaques associated with Alzheimer's disease. Over time, those plaques block cell-to-cell signaling. The plaques can also cause inflammation.

But supplementing with collagen, to boost the amount of type IV in the brain seems to stop amyloid-beta buildup and protect neurons from the toxic proteins.

Could Help Heal Gastrointestinal Issues

Like many of the tissues and muscles in your skin, your gastrointestinal (GI) tract relies on collagen for a great deal of its structure and maintenance. Digestive conditions like irritable bowel syndrome, inflammatory bowel disease, and leaky gut syndrome can cause inflammation and irritation along the GI tract, from your stomach to your bowels. If your body doesn't have enough collagen to heal and restore your gut, symptoms of these disorders and others might be compounded.

What's more, having one of the conditions might mean you start at a collagen deficit. Indeed, one study looked at the collagen levels of one hundred seventy patients with an inflammatory bowel disease. Half had ulcerative colitis (an inflammatory disease of the colon), and the other half had Crohn's disease. In these patients, serum levels of collagen were low. Therefore, researchers believe eating more collagen-rich foods or taking collagen supplements might help restore some of the much-needed collagen to GI tract muscles, which may in turn reduce inflammation and invite healing. Still, more research is needed to know how strong the connection is.

May Ease Back Pain

It stands to reason that a protein that has been found to prevent or ease painful joints and help bones sustain their strength might also play a pivotal role in easing back pain. However, few studies have looked at this exact affliction and the potential effects that collagen peptides or collagen-rich foods might have on it.

One study did find promising signs: researchers gave two hundred individuals, all age fifty or older, 1,200 milligrams of collagen hydrolysate or a placebo product every day for six months. At the six-month mark, participants that had been taking the collagen reported significantly less back pain compared to the placebo group. However, at a three-month checkpoint, there was no such difference. This result might point to the fact that the benefits of collagen are cumulative—you need to use it continuously for a period of time to see some of its benefits.

Could Restore Hair Loss

Cracking or splitting nails could be a result of low collagen, as could brittle hair that won't grow. Not only is collagen the building-block protein of bones, muscles, ligaments, and teeth, it's also the foundation of health for your nails and hair. Taking collagen may also increase hair strength and prevent strands from appearing weak or lifeless.

One study suggests that the extracellular matrix, which is made with collagen and helps support collagen structures throughout the body, may play a role in hair follicle regeneration. Future research is needed to confirm whether supplementing the diet with collagen can help restore hair loss.

Fast Facts

Collagen remains an area of interest in medical research because little is known about many of the impacts this protein has on health, wellness, and disease care. However, early and preliminary data reveal that collagen may be able to prevent or slow dementia, help heal diseases of the gastrointestinal tract, ease back pain, and even restore hair.

COLLAGEN-RICH FOODS

Collagen is found naturally in animal proteins, like beef, chicken, and fish. Its highest concentrations are in the connective tissues, including skin, bones, ligaments, and tendons.

Your body makes collagen for your most fundamental needs—building bones, strengthening muscles, and protecting joints. More collagen, however, can be a good thing. As we've learned, an aging body produces less and less collagen, so supplementing with collagen-rich foods and collagen supplements may boost the amounts of protein in your tissues, bones, and joints.

Currently, it's unclear how well the body absorbs collagen from food sources. Collagen cells, when coming straight from food, are quite large, and the body isn't particularly effective at using those to your benefit.

Collagen supplements, however, have been processed to make the collagen easier to absorb. Research supports the idea that using supplements can increase your collagen and encourage your body's own collagen production. It's unclear as yet if food is as beneficial.

With that being said, many of the most collagen-rich foods happen to be great for your body in a multitude of ways. Adding these foods to your diet might give you more collagen and can definitely provide other minerals, vitamins, and protein.

Bone Broth

You might not fancy sitting down to a meal of roasted tendon, cartilage, and bones, but simmering those tissues for long periods of time will render collagen, amino acids, gelatin, and a lot of delicious flavor. This concoction is known as bone broth.

Bone broth may be a trendy sipping beverage these days, but its potential impact on health has been known in alternative medicine circles for centuries. (Think the feel-good power of a bowl of chicken noodle soup, but better.)

Bone broth bars are popping up in America's largest cities. Perhaps the first and most widely heralded is Chef Marco Canora's Brodo, located in New York City. The restaurant began by serving piping-hot broth from a tiny window in the East Village. Today, Brodo has multiple locations across New York City and has inspired a plethora of bone broth enthusiasts to start similar ventures across the country.

If you don't have a neighborhood bone broth spot, you can make your own bone broth (see recipes pages **xxx** and **xxx**). You can also buy bone broth premade in frozen form and as capsules, bars, and powders.

Bone Marrow

Bone marrow is a spongy tissue that fills the center portion of large bones like the spine, hips, and thighs. It's rich in many vitamins and minerals, as well as in collagen.

Bone marrow was once consumed widely as part of the whole-animal approach to our ancestors' diet style, but it largely fell out of use. That is, until recently. With the renaissance of the whole-animal movement, the Paleo diet, and the nose-to-tail cooking style, chefs have returned bone marrow to restaurant menus, often as a high-priced option. (Just think: all those bones were once discarded and now we pay top dollar for them.)

But bone marrow isn't something you should put on the menu every night. It's fairly high in fat (12 grams in 1 tablespoon) and calories (110 per tablespoon)—measurements that are equivalent to a tablespoon of butter or oil. Bone marrow can also be difficult to source, or at least high-quality bones are. Restaurants often pay butchers directly for the best pieces, so you'll need to make friends with one to get some marrow if you're eager to try it.

Poultry

Many collagen supplements are made from chicken—both skin and bones—so it shouldn't come as a surprise that the barnyard fowl is a good source of collagen. Other forms of poultry, like turkeys, are a good source of collagen, too. Smaller birds—quails, for example—are less plentiful in the protein. Chicken is the primary source for collagen in the poultry group. If you take apart a whole chicken, you may notice how much connective tissue the bird has. Most of it turns supple when cooked, leaving almost every element but the bones edible—if you're willing, that is.

All of those tissues are a good source of collagen, so don't be shy about using up every bit of a chicken or turkey when you have one. One study found that chicken necks and cartilage (the tissues in joints) are especially good sources of collagen. A good butcher can save you these parts of a chicken or turkey for making your own broth.

Eggs

This quintessential breakfast food is an easy source of collagen building blocks. The yolk and white contain some of the essential amino acids, and the eggshell membrane does as well. (You don't need to crunch on shell to get the collagen, though; just add them to your next batch of bone broth.)

Eggs also contain an important trace mineral called sulfur. Sulfur is a required element of collagen production, so making sure your diet has enough is another way to boost collagen production and keep quantities high.

Fish and Shellfish

Just as poultry and cows have a great deal of collagen in their skin and bones, so do fish and shellfish. Marine collagen, or collagen derived from marine animals, is sold as its own supplement, and research suggests it might have beneficial impacts for heart health that other collagens have yet to show.

For the most collagen benefit, you'll need to think past filets and prime cuts. Most of the collagen in seafood and fish is in their skin, bones, scales, and head. In fact, those are the parts of the fish that are used to make marine collagen peptides. If you can't get down with gnawing on fish skin—some can be delicious when seared crispy—consider using high-quality fish bones to make a fish stock or broth, just as you might use beef and poultry bones to make bone broth.

Fast Facts

Some of the most collagen-rich foods may already be plentiful in your diet. Chicken, eggs, and fish can supply the protein, as can beef and bone marrow. If you need these collagen-rich parts for homemade broth or recipes, talk with your butcher. Many will be happy to save the best elements for you.

COLLAGEN-BOOSTING FOODS

In addition to foods that have their own collagen, many more foods actually help your body *make* more collagen or support its development. Most of them also happen to be incredibly good sources of vitamins, minerals, and antioxidants that have multiple benefits for the many conditions or issues you might be seeking to treat with collagen.

Want to improve signs of aging? The antioxidant form of vitamin A, beta-carotene, is found in carrots, sweet potatoes, and squash and can help erase damage caused by the sun's harmful ultraviolet (UV) rays. Vitamin E, an antioxidant found in abundance in almonds, can also neutralize the damage your skin takes from free radicals. Vitamin C is a vital link that makes collagen production happen. All of these also happen to have many other healthful benefits above and beyond their support of collagen.

So in addition to taking supplements or eating collagen-rich foods on the regular, you can do your body—and your skin, joints, bones, heart, and other elements—even more good by making sure you incorporate these foods into your diet, too.

Almonds

In addition to being a good source of protein and healthy fats, almonds happen to have an abundance of vitamin E, an antioxidant that is necessary for healthy skin and skin protection. Vitamin E also works with vitamin C to stimulate collagen formation.

What's more, almonds are a good source of copper, an essential trace element that research says is necessary for the final formation of collagen fibrils. Other nuts and seeds, like sunflower seeds, cashews, and Brazil nuts, are also good sources of both vitamin E and copper.

Broccoli

These petite, green, treelike vegetables are a solid source of vitamin C. Vitamin C is an essential part of collagen formation. It's found in the outer layer of skin, the epidermis, and it helps regulate the production of procollagen, a precursor to collagen. Your body cannot make vitamin C, so it must have it from food or supplements. Plus, your body cannot make collagen without vitamin C, so it's necessary to make sure you have enough in order to keep collagen production running smoothly.

You can actually get a good deal of your recommended daily value of vitamin C in just one serving of broccoli. A half-cup of cooked broccoli has 51 milligrams of vitamin C. The recommended daily goal for men is 90 milligrams; for women, it's 75 milligrams. So one serving nets more than half for men and almost three-quarters for women. (Pregnant and nursing women need more vitamin C: 85 milligrams if you're pregnant and 120 milligrams if you're nursing.)

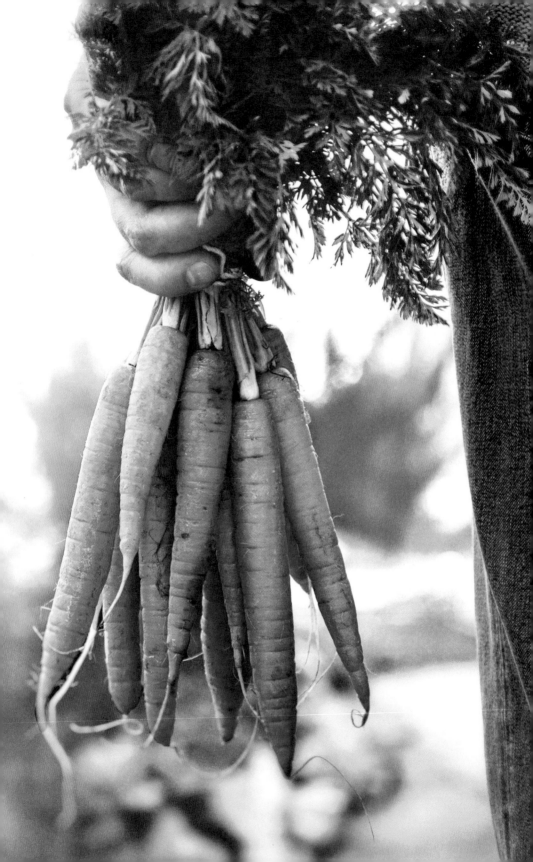

Carrots

Carrots—and other orange vegetables and fruits like sweet potatoes, pumpkin, cantaloupe, apricots, squash, and mango—contain carotenoids, a type of vitamin A. (Oranges, interestingly enough, do not have vitamin A.) Vitamin A is integral to healthy skin. It boosts collagen production, removes dead cells in the upper layers of your skin, and encourages cell renewal.

Topical vitamin A treatments, including serums and antiaging creams, have been shown to boost collagen production and reduce signs of aging, like wrinkles and fine lines. Getting plenty of vitamin A in your diet is a good way to make sure you are not deficient and that your body can maintain its healthy collagen-production process.

Adult men should aim for 900 micrograms of vitamin A per day; women need 700 micrograms unless pregnant or lactating. In that case, they need more—770 micrograms is the recommended dietary allowance for pregnant women, and 1300 micrograms for lactating women. Thankfully, delicious foods like carrots and squash help you get all the vitamin A you need. One cup of raw carrot strips contains 459 micrograms. One baked sweet potato has more than 1,400 micrograms.

Citrus Fruits

Lemons, limes, oranges, and grapefruits—they're good for more than a beautiful centerpiece at your next dinner party. These citrus fruits are rich in vitamin C, the water-soluble vitamin and antioxidant that is vital to collagen production.

They also happen to be at their peak in winter months: November through March. That's precisely when so many other good sources of vitamin C—berries, tomatoes, peppers, and more—aren't. Be aware that if you're buying those, they're certainly unlikely to be grown locally. Give your thanks to nature for knowing exactly what we need to get through the long, dark days of winter.

SCURVY AT SEA:
WHAT PIRATES AND SAILORS
HAVE TO DO WITH COLLAGEN

Vitamin C, also known as L-ascorbic acid, is an essential water-soluble vitamin. It's crucial to many of the body's most important functions, from metabolizing protein for energy to limiting the impact of dangerous free radicals on the body's cells.

But as essential as vitamin C is to so many physical processes, the human body cannot make vitamin C on its own. It must instead get the antioxidant from dietary sources, which include citrus fruits, broccoli, peppers, and Brussels sprouts.

These foods aren't particularly shelf-stable, which means they were unlikely to be carried aboard eighteenth-century ships. For sailors, pirates, and others aboard boats, a life at sea without vitamin C could be a dangerous life indeed.

As vitamin C levels drop, the body cannot convert procollagen (the collagen precursor) into collagen as well as it should. That means collagen strands don't form and fibrils can't assemble into the incredibly strong triple helices that make up collagen's cellular construction. As a result, connective tissues weaken, and joint pain, swelling, and poor wound healing may be noticed. As the deficiency worsens, gums may bleed easily and teeth may fall out. Iron-deficiency anemia may develop, with increased bleeding. Ultimately, this deficiency of vitamin C, called scurvy, can be deadly.

Sailors who set sail in the eighteenth century certainly knew about the risks of scurvy, but it wasn't until the mid-eighteenth century that British navy surgeon Sir James Lind discovered that oranges, and citrus fruits in general, could stop scurvy.

He recommended that members of the British navy eat fresh citrus fruits and drink lemon juice to ward off the disease.

It took nearly two more centuries for researchers to understand that ascorbic acid—the word *ascorbus* means "no scurvy"—was the key to keeping seafaring folk healthy and well. That's when Dr. Albert Szent-Györgyi of Budapest isolated the vitamin C molecule in a red pepper and discovered the role it played in scurvy. He won the Nobel Prize in Physiology or Medicine in 1937 for this discovery.

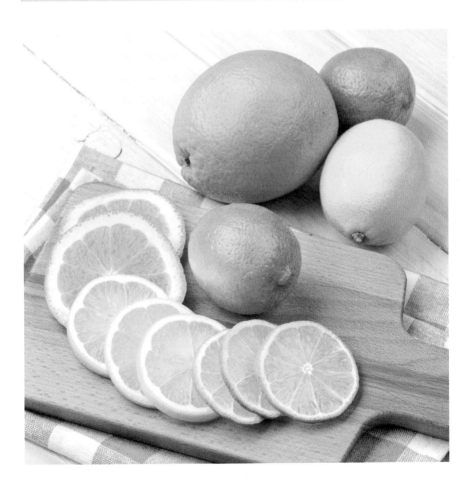

Eggs

Eggs—yolks and whites—are important to collagen production. The whites contain the amino acids glycine and proline, which are building blocks of collagen. But the whole egg is worth the seventy or so calories. It packs healthy fats, high-quality protein, and a bit of sulfur, too.

Garlic

Those pungent bulbs that boost the flavor of everything from omelets to beef stew contain a mineral called sulfur. Sulfur is thought to help ramp up the body's collagen synthesis process. What's more, garlic contains an amino acid called taurine that has been shown to help support and remake damaged collagen fibers.

Kiwi

Like berries, the kiwifruit—and its smaller counterpart, kiwi berries— are potent sources of vitamin C, a necessary component of pre-collagen production.

Some studies suggest that vitamin C may help erase photodamage caused by the sun's UV rays and skin aging caused by free radicals. Exposure to the sun can destroy collagen and slow collagen production. Vitamin C may help restore that healthy cycle. Vitamin C also speeds up wound-healing by increasing collagen synthesis so that the skin has more of the cells and strands it needs to heal and recover.

Leafy Green Vegetables

Popeye the Sailor knew his spinach would make him grow strong, but he may not have realized his love for the leafy greens probably also resulted in healthier joints and younger-looking skin. Leafy greens like spinach, kale, and turnip greens are brimming with vitamins C, E, and A. All of these vitamins are essential parts of the collagen synthesis process in the body. Plus, each has its own benefits for reducing many related conditions, from skin aging to free radical damage.

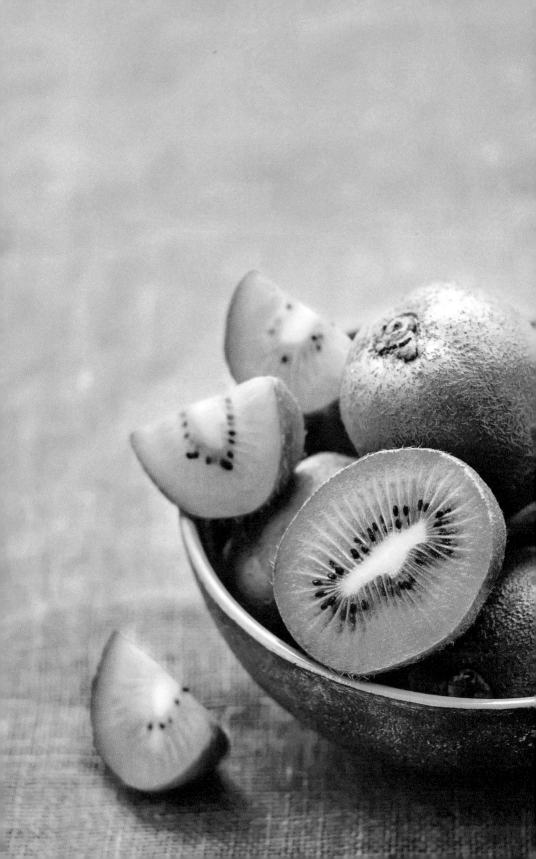

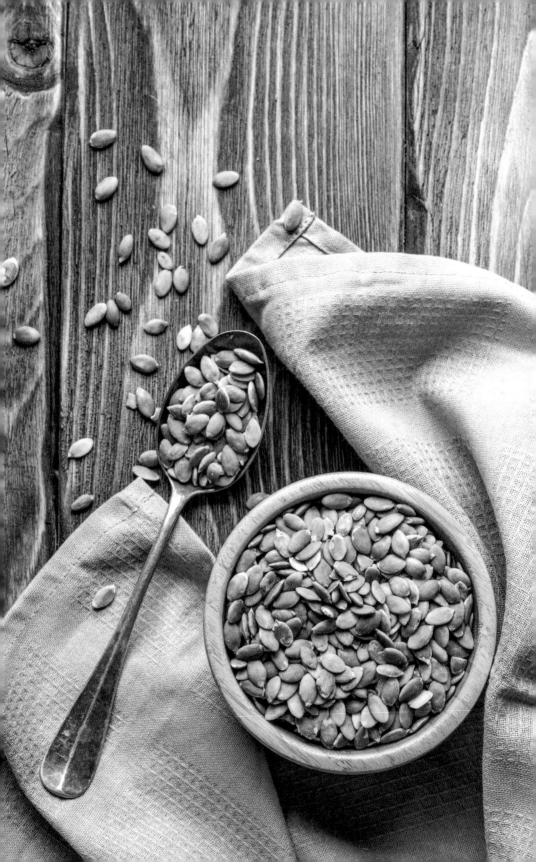

Oysters

If you're searching for zinc, your hunt is over. Oysters contain more zinc than any other food. Though you probably won't be snacking on half-shells every day, it's A-OK to throw back a half dozen or so any time you get the opportunity. Three ounces of oysters contains 74 milligrams of zinc. That's 493 percent of your daily value.

In addition to increasing collagen production, zinc is essential for bone formation, and bone is made up of collagen, too. When you are zinc deficient, your bones cannot make new cells as efficiently. Being low on zinc can also slow wound-healing. Having enough zinc in your diet encourages cell turnover and collagen production, which speeds up the healing of cuts, wounds, and other skin damage.

Other proteins—red meat and poultry—actually provide the majority of zinc to the American diet. But fish and seafood are typically a good source. For example, Alaskan crab has 6.5 milligrams in three ounces. Three ounces of lobster has almost one-quarter of the daily value, with 3.4 milligrams.

Pumpkin Seeds

Zinc, a trace element found in pumpkin seeds, is a collagen cofactor. That means it activates all the proteins and amino acids that are necessary for the production of collagen. A 1-ounce serving of pumpkin seeds has 2.9 milligrams, or about 19 percent of your recommended daily value

Pumpkin seeds, or pepitas, aren't the only seeds that are a good source of zinc. In fact, some seeds have even more zinc. Hemp seeds, for instance, contain 21 percent of the average daily value in 1 ounce. (One ounce is about 1 tablespoon.) One ounce of pine nuts has 1.8 milligrams, or about 12 percent of your daily goal.

Strawberries

These ruby-red berries are a great source of vitamin C, or ascorbic acid. If you like other berries—blueberries, raspberries, or blackberries—you're in luck. These berries are also filled with the powerful antioxidant, can help protect against signs of skin aging and skin damage, and encourage collagen production. All of them can also help you get more protein into your body.

Fast Facts

Eating collagen-rich foods isn't every element of the equation. In order to help your body properly produce and use collagen, you need to fill your diet with foods rich in particular vitamins and minerals, like vitamin C, vitamin A, and vitamin E. The good news is, many of these vitamins are found in foods that are already part of the typical American diet.

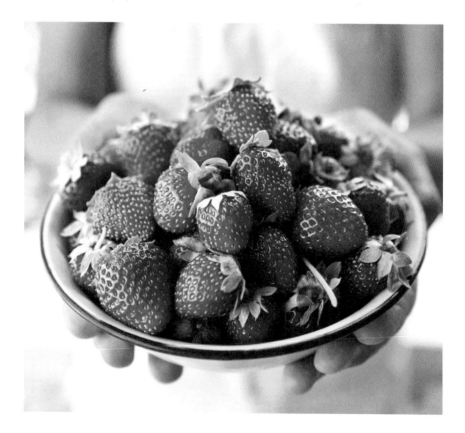

SHOULD I TAKE A VITAMIN C SUPPLEMENT?

Humans cannot make their own vitamin C. Every bit of the vitamin you get must come from your diet. However, your body doesn't absorb every milligram of the water-soluble vitamin you take in.

Approximately 70 to 90 percent of vitamin C is absorbed at doses between 30 and 180 milligrams per day. That's a moderate dose, considering the daily recommended value is 90 milligrams for men and 75 milligrams for women. (Pregnant or nursing mothers should get more.)

However, if you try to take even more, the absorption rate falls. At a daily dose of 1 gram of vitamin C, only about 50 percent of the antioxidant is absorbed. The rest is removed from your body through urine.

It is possible, though unlikely, to get too much vitamin C. Excessive doses of the vitamin aren't typically problematic. You may experience gastrointestinal issues like diarrhea, bloating, and abdominal cramps. If you have a history of kidney stones, know that high vitamin C intake can increase urinary oxalate, which can contribute to kidney stone formation.

But vitamin C is abundant in so many easily accessible foods—citrus fruits, kiwifruit, bell peppers, broccoli, tomatoes, etc. The likelihood that anyone will be vitamin C deficient is slim. Most people will be able to get everything they need from their diet.

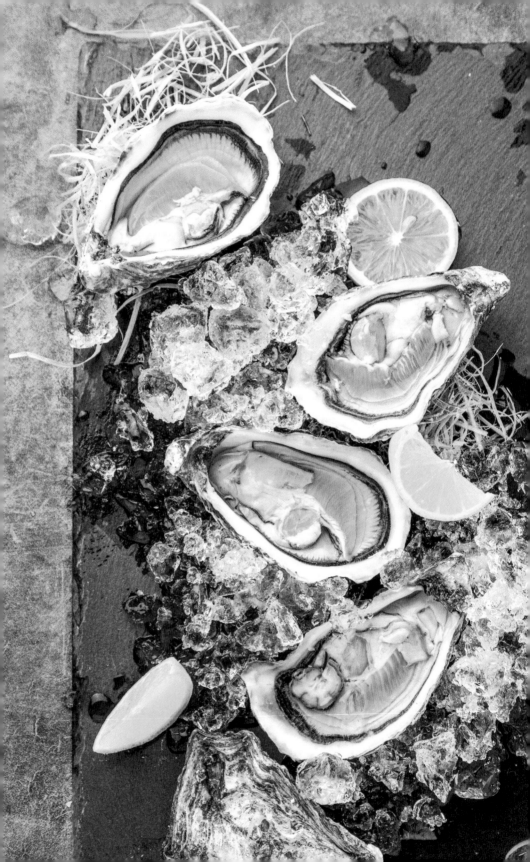

PART 3

Collagen Recipes

Cooking with collagen-rich foods or collagen supplements provides an opportunity to boost your natural collagen network and improve your overall health. Many collagen-rich foods, including eggs and bone broth, happen to be incredibly comforting and delicious. Collagen supplements can be flavorless, which means they're great for putting into any number of dishes. Companies also produce collagen supplements and peptides with unique and distinctive flavors that make them especially fun for a variety of dishes.

In its hydrolysate form, collagen is a source of protein (about 18 grams in a 20-gram serving) that should be factored into your daily nutritional goals. However, it isn't a particularly impactful source of calories—one 20-gram serving of unflavored collagen peptides has just 70 calories—which allows you a bit more freedom to use it in a variety of ways without worrying about significantly impacting your daily caloric intake.

The recipes in this chapter were chosen because they are delicious and fun and because they incorporate collagen and gelatin in ways that pair protein-boosting foods with other beneficial vitamins and minerals.

The recipes in this chapter were chosen because they are delicious and fun and because they incorporate collagen and gelatin in ways that pair protein-boosting foods with other beneficial vitamins and minerals. If you're new to incorporating collagen into your meals and snacks, start with dishes you're already familiar with—soups, stews, and brothy noodle dishes. If you've been eating collagen for a while or using supplements, have some fun with the slushes, gummies, and shakes.

Everyone can benefit from keeping collagen-infused water on hand, too, so don't leave home without it.

SWEET POTATO-GREENS HASH

Start your day with a hash of sweet potato cubes and silky sautéed greens (all the vitamin C you'll need!). As a bonus, the fried egg serves up high-quality protein and amino acids that are vital to collagen production.

Makes 4 servings

WHAT YOU'LL NEED:

3¼ tablespoons olive oil, divided

1 small red onion, peeled and vertically sliced

2 cloves garlic, chopped

5 cups peeled cubed sweet potatoes

¼ cup water

5 packed cups baby kale, baby spinach, or a combination (about 5 ounces)

¾ teaspoon kosher salt

½ teaspoon freshly ground black pepper

4 eggs

4 teaspoons hot sauce (optional)

WHAT YOU'LL DO:

1. Heat a large skillet over medium-high heat. Add 2 tablespoons olive oil to the pan; swirl to coat. Add the onion; cook for 5 minutes or until tender. Add the garlic to the pan and cook 1 minute, or until lightly browned, stirring constantly. Add the potatoes and water. Cover and cook over medium heat for 12–15 minutes, or until the potatoes are tender and easily pierced with a fork, stirring every 4 minutes. Stir in the leafy greens, salt, and pepper.

2. Heat another medium skillet over medium heat. Add the remaining 1 tablespoon oil to the pan; swirl to coat. Break 2 eggs into the pan; cook for 3–4 minutes, or until the eggs reach your desired degree of doneness. Carefully remove the eggs, then cook the remaining 2 eggs.

3. Divide the hash among four plates. Top each with 1 egg and drizzle with hot sauce, if desired.

COCONUT COLLAGEN OATMEAL

For its creaminess, this oatmeal recipe uses deeply nourishing coconut manna, a coconut spread that can be used in place of butter and cream.

Makes 2 servings

WHAT YOU'LL NEED:

2 cups water

1 cup rolled oats

2 tablespoons coconut manna

1 scoop collagen peptides

1 teaspoon honey

Dash of ground cinnamon

Pinch of nutmeg

Pinch of kosher salt

Strawberries, cacao nibs, and toasted coconut chips (for garnish)

WHAT YOU'LL DO:

1. Bring the water to a boil. Add the oats; cook according to package directions.

2. When the oats are cooked, stir in the coconut manna, peptides, honey, cinnamon, nutmeg, and salt. Simmer until the manna is melted and absorbed.

3. Divide into two servings. Top with strawberries, cacao nibs, coconut chips, or other toppings of your choice.

COLLAGEN-PACKED BLUEBERRY MUFFINS

Start your morning with a hearty dose of filling protein thanks to these muffins. Juicy blueberries stud each baked muffin for a burst of tart-sweetness and collagen-boosting vitamin C.

Makes 6 muffins

WHAT YOU'LL NEED:

4½ scoops unflavored collagen peptides

1 cup white whole-wheat flour

½ cup stevia-erythritol blend or 1 cup coconut sugar

2 teaspoons baking powder

½ teaspoon kosher salt

1 egg

3 egg whites

¼ cup creamy sunflower or almond butter

¼ cup unsweetened vanilla oat milk or unsweetened vanilla almond milk

2 tablespoons coconut oil

1 teaspoon vanilla extract

1 cup fresh blueberries

WHAT YOU'LL DO:

1. Preheat oven to 350°F. In a large mixing bowl, combine the peptides, flour, stevia-erythritol blend, baking powder, and salt. Create a well in the center of the dry ingredients.

2. In a medium mixing bowl, combine the egg, egg whites, sunflower butter, oat milk, coconut oil, and vanilla extract. Pour this wet mixture into the well of dry ingredients. Fold together until just moistened. Add the blueberries and gently fold to evenly disperse throughout the batter.

3. Coat the wells of a six-muffin pan with a light spray of cooking oil, or use paper muffin liners. Divide the muffin batter evenly among the wells. Bake at 350°F for 20–25 minutes, or until a toothpick inserted in the middle comes out clean. Cool the muffins in the pan for 5 minutes, then remove from the pan and let cool completely on a wire rack. Store in an airtight container in the fridge for up to 4 days.

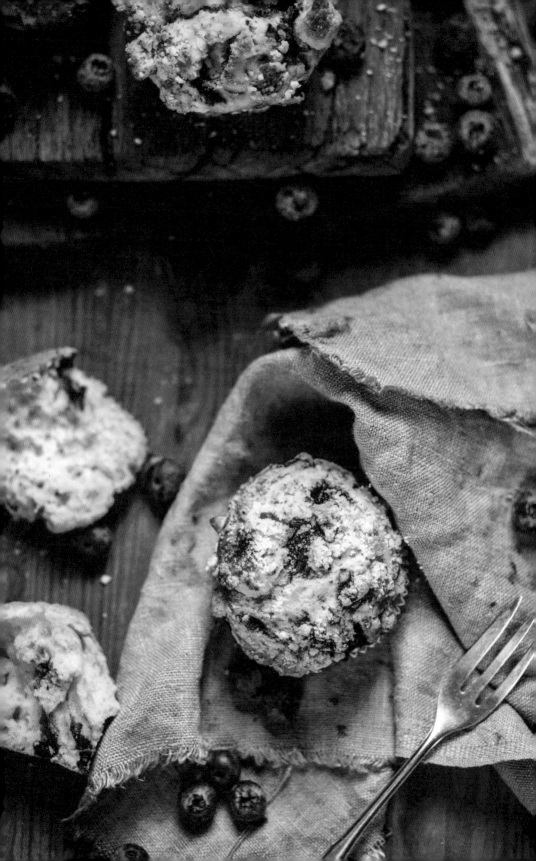

TRIPLE-BERRY COLLAGEN OVERNIGHT OATS

The beauty of overnight oats is that the moment your eyes pop open in the morning, your breakfast is complete. You can also get creative once you understand the basic ratios and make just about any combination of ingredients you want. This is a beginner recipe, but don't be shy about trying new ingredients. If you don't like it, tomorrow is a new day—and a new batch of overnight oats.

Makes 1 serving

WHAT YOU'LL NEED:

- ½ cup rolled oats
- 1 cup vanilla kefir or drinkable yogurt (such as Siggi's)
- 1 tablespoon unsweetened vanilla oat milk
- 1 scoop unflavored collagen peptides
- Dash of cinnamon
- ½ cup frozen three-berry mixture

WHAT YOU'LL DO:

1. In a mason jar or other hard-sided container with a sealable lid, add the oats, kefir, milk, peptides, and cinnamon. Stir until well combined. Top with frozen berries. Refrigerate overnight, or for at least 8 hours.

2. Before eating, stir to break up the berries and combine them with the oat mixture. If the oats are too thick, add 1 tablespoon oat milk until you reach your desired consistency.

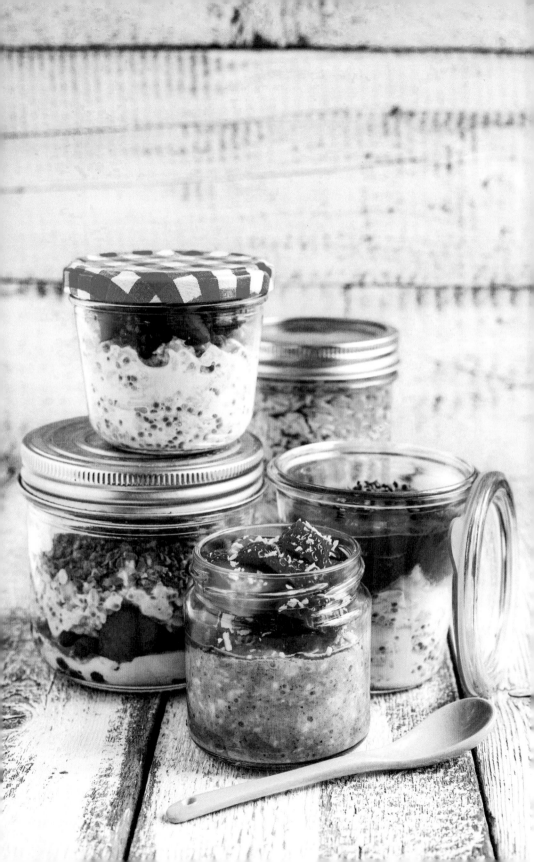

OVERNIGHT OAT INGREDIENT MATH

You can make any combination of ingredients you like for your overnight oats as long as you get the oats-to-liquid ratio correct. It's a 2-to-1 ratio of milk or yogurt to rolled oats. You'll need an extra splash of oat milk (2 tablespoons) to account for the collagen peptides, too.

With that math in mind, you can make any combination you please. The following combinations are included here to provide inspiration:

PEACH-BLUEBERRY COLLAGEN OVERNIGHT OATS

1. Top the oat mixture with 1 peach, seeded and chopped; ¼ cup blueberries; and 2 tablespoons toasted walnuts. Serves 1.

TIP: Don't put crunchy toppings, such as nuts, in your oat mixture until just before eating.

PEANUT BUTTER CUP COLLAGEN OVERNIGHT OATS

1. Stir 1 tablespoon peanut butter into the oat mixture. (You may need an extra tablespoon of oat milk in the morning.) Before eating, top with 1 tablespoon mini dark chocolate chips or 1 tablespoon chopped dark chocolate. Serves 1.

APPLE PIE COLLAGEN OVERNIGHT OATS

1. Stir 1 tablespoon maple syrup, a dash of nutmeg, and 1 tablespoon chia seeds into the oat mixture. Top with ½ large apple, grated. Stir to combine. Before eating, top with 2 tablespoons toasted walnuts or pecans. Serves 1.

MATCHA COLLAGEN OVERNIGHT OATS

1. Stir 1 tablespoon matcha and 1 tablespoon chia seeds into the oat mixture. (You may need an extra tablespoon of oat milk in the morning.) Before eating, top with 1 tablespoon unsweetened shredded coconut. Serves 1.

STRAWBERRY-BANANA COLLAGEN OVERNIGHT OATS

1. Stir 2 teaspoons strawberry preserves into the oat mixture, then top with ⅓ cup frozen strawberries. Before eating, stir strawberries into the oat mixture and top with ½ banana, sliced. Serves 1.

OATMEAL BANANA PANCAKES

Brunch is better with collagen-rich pancakes. If you don't want to use maple syrup, serve with a drizzle of warmed peanut butter or strawberry syrup.

Makes 2 servings

WHAT YOU'LL NEED:

⅔ cup oat flour

1 banana, mashed

¼ cup unsweetened oat milk

1 large egg

2 scoops unflavored collagen peptides

½ teaspoon pure vanilla extract

¼ teaspoon ground cinnamon

3 large egg whites

WHAT YOU'LL DO:

1. Combine the oat flour, banana, oat milk, egg, peptides, vanilla extract, and cinnamon until just moistened.

2. Whip the egg whites until foamy. Then gently fold them into the pancake batter.

3. Preheat a griddle or large nonstick skillet. Coat the pan with oil or melted butter, swirling to coat. Spoon about 2½ tablespoons batter per pancake onto the griddle. Cook for 2–3 minutes, or until the tops are covered in bubbles. Flip and cook for another 2–3 minutes, or until lightly browned.

STOVETOP BONE BROTH

Bone broth may be as close as you can get to the magic of a witch's brew. But instead of potions and spells, you're stirring up an enriched stock that's full of healing collagen, vitamins, and minerals.

Making bone broth is a labor of love, no matter how you make it. You can give yourself a bit of a head start on the process by saving vegetable scraps (carrot peels, onion skins, celery leaves, etc.) and chicken or beef bones and freezing them until you're ready to simmer and boil yourself a hearty pot of bone broth.

Makes about 8 cups

WHAT YOU'LL NEED:

- 3 pounds chicken bones
- 1 head garlic, unpeeled and halved horizontally
- 1 large onion, skin-on, quartered
- 2 medium carrots, unpeeled, chopped
- 2 stalks celery, chopped
- 2 bay leaves
- 1 tablespoon whole black peppercorns
- 2 tablespoons apple cider vinegar
- Water

WHAT YOU'LL DO:

1. Preheat oven to 450°F. Line a rimmed baking sheet with aluminum foil or parchment paper. Rinse the bones and pat dry. Arrange the bones on a baking sheet along with the garlic.

2. Roast for 20 minutes. Remove the sheet pan from the oven and add the onion and carrots. Roast for another 20 minutes, or until browned.

3. Transfer the bones and vegetables to a large stockpot (at least 6-quart capacity). Add the celery, bay leaves, peppercorns, and vinegar. Add enough water to fill the stockpot (about 12 cups). Cover and let rest for 20 minutes.

4. Bring the broth to a rapid simmer over medium-high heat. Reduce the heat to low and place the lid slightly ajar. Occasionally skim any foam and excess fat from the surface through the first hour.

5. After the first hour, securely place the lid on the stockpot and let it cook for at least 10 additional hours, but up to 24 hours. Add more water occasionally to keep the bones and vegetables fully submerged during the cooking process.

NOTE: Do not leave broth unattended on a hot stove. You can cool the pot and store it in your fridge, then bring it back to simmering the next day.

6. When the broth is at your desired flavor and color (look for a rich golden color for chicken or a deep umber for beef), remove the stockpot from the stovetop and let it cool slightly. Strain the broth through a fine-mesh sieve or a cheesecloth-lined colander. Discard the bones and vegetables.

7. Fill a sink, tub, or very large pot with ice. Place the broth in its container into the ice. Stir the broth frequently to reduce its temperature. When the broth is lukewarm, divide it among sealable containers, cover, and immediately refrigerate. The next day, scoop any solidified fat from the broth's surface.

STORAGE: You can store the broth in a fridge for up to 5 days or freeze it for up to 3 months.

BEEF OR CHICKEN?

Beef bone broth usually earns the most fans thanks to its rich and intense flavor, but you'll find no arguments against chicken bone broth here. The broth (and that good-as-gold gelatinous fat) will bring immense flavor to soups, stews, and more.

WHICH BONES ARE BEST?

If you're using chicken bones, make sure you have a mix of breast, back, and wing bones. The latter two have more collagen-rich marrow, which boosts your brew's flavor and collagen count.

If you're using beef bones, try a combination of large roast or sholder bones and smaller bones, like those in the neck or ribs. Be sure to ask your local butcher for quality bones. Most would be thrilled to keep them out of the trash heap.

CAN YOU KEEP THE SOLIDIFIED FAT FROM BONE BROTH?

Yes, the solidified fat that rises to the top of broth as it cools is useable, but it will spoil quickly if you don't handle it properly.

To keep bone broth fat for later use, you'll need to cook off all the liquid. This will leave you with just the solid fat. If you don't have a lot of fat left over from your batch of broth, store it in the freezer and wait until you have more after a second, or even a third, batch. This way you'll get a big reward for a good bit of work. Just be sure to defrost the fat before continuing with these next steps.

1. Place the fat in a slow cooker. Cook on LOW for 6 hours, with the lid slightly ajar to allow moisture evaporation.

2. Scoop all the liquefied fat into a jar and let it cool at room temperature without a lid for 1 hour. Then, seal the jar and store it in the fridge to cool completely. Use in place of ghee, butter, or other solid fats.

NOTE: In the fridge, the fat from bone broth will last several months.

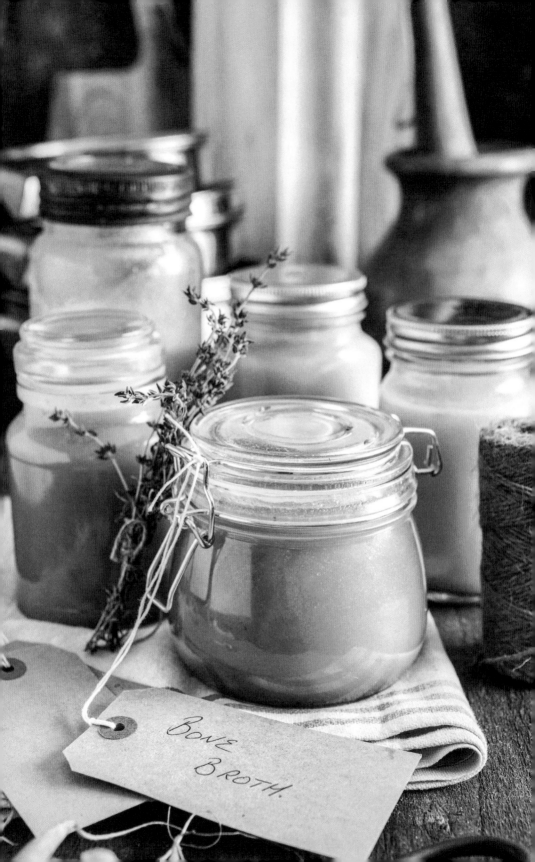

BONE
BROTH.

SLOW-COOKER BONE BROTH

If you live nowhere near a broth bar or just prefer making your own at home, you're in luck. A slow cooker works magic to turn large vats of bones, vegetable scraps, and water into liquid gold.

Makes 3–4 cups

WHAT YOU'LL NEED:

3½ pounds chicken or beef bones, oxtail, neck, ribs, or a combination

1 large yellow onion, skin-on, chopped

3 cloves garlic, smashed

3 carrots, chopped

2 stalks celery, chopped

Water

2 tablespoons apple cider vinegar

1 teaspoon kosher salt

3 teaspoons whole black peppercorns

WHAT YOU'LL DO:

1. Rinse and dry the bones. Set aside.

2. Place the onion, garlic, carrots, and celery in a 6-quart slow cooker. Add the bones. Add enough water to cover the bones. Stir in the vinegar, salt, and peppercorns.

3. Cook on LOW for 16–24 hours, or until the broth is golden brown and deeply aromatic.

4. Carefully pour the broth through a fine-mesh sieve into a large bowl or jug. Discard the solids.

5. Fill a sink, tub, or very large pot with ice. Place the broth in its container into the ice. Stir the broth frequently to reduce its temperature.

6. When the broth is lukewarm, divide it among sealable containers, cover, and immediately refrigerate. The next day, scoop any solidified fat from the broth's surface.

STORAGE: You can store the broth in the fridge for up to 5 days or freeze it for up to 3 months.

HOW TO FREEZE BONE BROTH

Most broth recipes will make several cups, a gracious plenty even for the most broth-thirsty. Freezing is a great way to save up for future meals or cold days.

WHAT YOU'LL NEED:

Silicone ice cube trays, preferably 2-inch square molds

Large zip-top bags

Permanent marker

WHAT TO DO:

* Once you've completely cooled the broth and removed any solidified fat from its surface, carefully pour the broth you're planning to freeze into ice cube tray molds. Freeze for at least 6 hours, or overnight.

* Remove each block of frozen bone broth from the mold and place it in a zip-top bag labeled with the date you made the broth.

* Use these small frozen cubes to prepare a bit of bone broth quickly. You can melt them into soups, stews, pastas, or rice dishes.

CHICKEN ZOODLE SOUP

If you make homemade broth, you'll have a lot to work with for several days. Put them to good use in comforting, filling dinners like this classic soup. To keep things lighter, use spiralized zucchini in place of flour-based pasta.

Makes 6 servings

WHAT YOU'LL NEED:

1½ pounds boneless, skinless chicken thighs, cut into bite-size pieces

1 teaspoon kosher salt

½ teaspoon freshly ground black pepper

1 tablespoon ghee, divided

1 cup diced yellow onion

1 cup chopped carrots

1 cup diced celery

2 cloves garlic, minced

2 teaspoons chopped oregano leaves

2 teaspoons chopped thyme leaves

5 cups chicken bone broth, homemade (page 82) or store-bought

3 zucchini squash, spiral-cut

Parsley, minced (for garnish)

WHAT YOU'LL DO:

1. Season the chicken pieces with the salt and pepper. Heat ½ tablespoon ghee in a medium Dutch oven over medium-high heat; swirl to coat. Sauté the chicken pieces until just browned. Remove the chicken from the Dutch oven and set aside.

2. Add the remaining ghee to the pan. Add the onion, carrots, and celery. Cook for 3–5 minutes, stirring occasionally. Add the garlic and cook 1 minute.

3. Return the cooked chicken to the Dutch oven. Add the oregano and thyme and stir to combine. Pour the bone broth over the chicken and vegetable mixture. Bring to a boil. When boiling, place the lid on the pan. Reduce the heat to medium-low. Simmer for 15 minutes.

4. Before serving, stir in the squash spirals. Let the zoodles sit for 3–5 minutes in the hot soup to soften. Garnish with parsley, if desired.

THAI COCONUT CHICKEN SOUP (TOM KHA GAI)

Use your homemade chicken bone broth or store-bought bone broth to bring rich, luscious flavor to dinner—ginger, lime, lemongrass, and delicately sweet coconut milk.

Makes 4 servings

WHAT YOU'LL NEED:

- 1 tablespoon olive oil or fat from homemade bone broth (page 78)
- 8 ounces cremini mushrooms, sliced
- 1 red pepper, sliced
- 1 shallot, cut horizontally into rounds
- 2 cloves garlic, minced
- 2 stalks lemongrass, cut into 1-inch pieces and crushed
- ¾ pound boneless, skinless chicken thighs, cut into 1-inch pieces

- 1 tablespoon Thai red chili paste (page 78)
- 3 cups chicken bone broth, homemade (page 82) or store-bought
- 1 (13.5-ounce) can coconut milk
- 1½ tablespoons fish sauce
- 6 quarter-size slices peeled ginger
- ¼ cup chopped fresh cilantro
- 1 lime, cut into wedges

WHAT YOU'LL DO:

1. Heat a large Dutch oven over medium-high heat. Add the oil to pan; swirl to coat. Add the mushrooms, red pepper, shallot, garlic, and lemongrass. Cook for 4 minutes, stirring occasionally.

2. Heat a medium nonstick skillet over medium-high heat. Add the chicken and cook for 5 minutes, or until the chicken is cooked through and no longer pink when cut open with a knife. Remove from the skillet and set aside.

3. Add the chili paste to the broth-vegetable mixture in the Dutch oven. Cook for 1 minute, stirring constantly. Add the bone broth, coconut milk, fish sauce, and ginger. Bring to a boil. Adjust the heat to low; let

simmer 10 minutes. Add the chicken to the soup. Cook for 2 minutes, or until heated through. Remove the ginger and lemongrass with a slotted spoon and discard. Divide among four bowls. Serve each bowl with a sprinkle of cilantro and a lime wedge.

TIP: Freeze extras in individual servings for a quick lunch or dinner down the road.

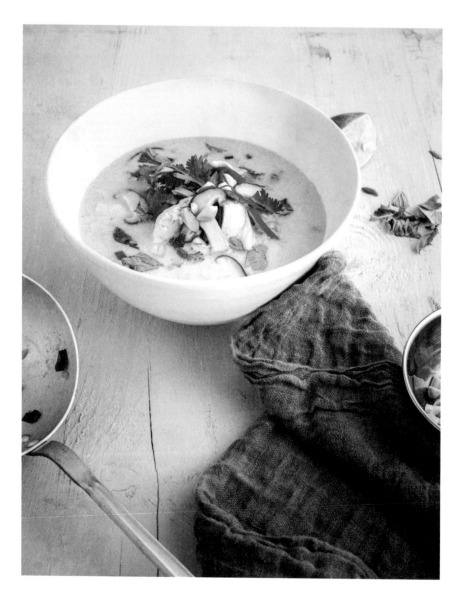

BONE BROTH RAMEN

Turn your long-cooked bone broth into an extra-special dinner that serves up several collagen-boosting ingredients in each helping.

Make 4 servings

WHAT YOU'LL NEED:

- 2 bundles (9.5 ounce) 100% buckwheat soba noodles
- 4 cups chicken or beef bone broth, homemade (page 78) or store-bought
- 3 cloves garlic, minced
- 6 quarter-size pieces of peeled ginger
- 1 cup shiitake mushrooms, sliced
- 2 cups baby bok choy
- 4 soft-boiled eggs
- 2 green onions, green parts chopped
- 4 teaspoons dark sesame oil
  Sriracha sauce and 1 lime, cut into wedges (optional)

WHAT YOU'LL DO:

1. Cook the soba noodles according to the package directions.

2. In a medium Dutch oven, heat the bone broth, garlic, ginger, mushrooms, and boy choy. Bring to a boil and cook for 4–5 minutes, or until the mushrooms are tender and the bok choy is wilted.

3. Remove the Dutch oven from heat. Remove the ginger pieces with a slotted spoon and discard. Divide the ramen among four bowls. Slice the eggs in half and arrange two halves in each bowl. Sprinkle with the green onions and drizzle with dark sesame oil. Top with sriracha and lime quarters, if desired.

COLLAGEN-RICH CLASSIC BEEF STEW

Increasing collagen in your favorite beef stew can be as simple as swapping regular beef broth for collagen-rich beef bone broth. You can also add beef collagen peptides for even more of the protein.

Makes 6 servings

WHAT YOU'LL NEED:

- 2 tablespoons canola oil, divided
- 1¼ pounds boneless chuck roast, or similar lean beef stew cut, cubed
- 1 medium yellow onion, peeled and chopped
- 3 tablespoons whole-wheat flour
- 3½ cups beef bone broth, homemade (page 78) or store-bought
- 1 cup dry red wine
- 2 tablespoons tomato paste
- 1½ cups chopped carrots (about 3 medium)
- 1 cup chopped celery (about 3 stalks)
- 1 pound Yukon gold potatoes, cubed
- 1½ cups water
- 3 thyme sprigs
- 1 bay leaf
- 1 teaspoon kosher salt
- ½ teaspoon freshly ground black pepper

WHAT YOU'LL DO:

1. Heat a large Dutch oven over medium-high heat. Add 2 teaspoons oil; swirl to coat. Add half the beef; cook for 5 minutes, or until browned, stirring occasionally. Remove the beef from the Dutch oven and set aside. Heat 2 teaspoons oil; swirl to coat. Cook the remaining beef for 5 minutes, or until browned, stirring occasionally. Remove the remaining beef from the Dutch oven and set aside.

2. Heat the remaining 2 teaspoons of oil in the Dutch oven; swirl to coat. Add the onion and sauté for 2 minutes.

3. In a separate bowl, add the flour to the bone broth; whisk until fully combined. Add the flour-bone broth mixture to the onion in the Dutch oven. Place the beef back in the Dutch oven, then add the red wine and the next seven ingredients (through the bay leaf). Bring to a

boil. Reduce the heat to low and let simmer, uncovered, for 45 minutes, stirring occasionally. When the beef is cooked and the potatoes are tender, add the salt and pepper. Stir, and let sit for 5 minutes. Remove the thyme sprigs and bay leaf with a slotted spoon and discard.

4. Divide the stew among six bowls to serve.

TIP: If you don't have wine, you can use additional bone broth.

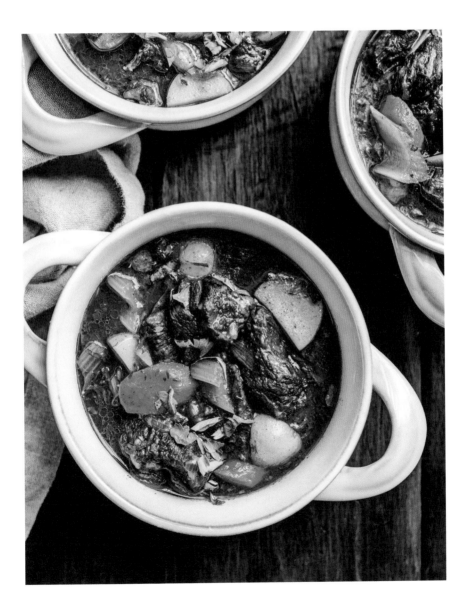

SWEET POTATO SOUP WITH COLLAGEN

Sweet potato is one of the richest sources of vitamin A in the modern diet. A bowlful of this luscious soup will provide you with all the beta-carotene you need.

Makes 4 servings

WHAT YOU'LL NEED:

- 3 pounds sweet potatoes, halved lengthwise
- 1 tablespoon olive oil
- 1 yellow onion, peeled and chopped
- 3 cloves garlic, chopped
- ½ teaspoon ground cumin
- ⅛ teaspoon ground red pepper
- ¼ teaspoon ground white pepper
- ½ teaspoon kosher salt

- 4 cups chicken bone broth, homemade (page 78) or store-bought
- 2 scoops unflavored collagen peptides
- 4 slices bacon, cooked and crumbled; 1 ounce shaved pecorino Romano cheese;
- 1 tablespoon minced fresh chives (optional)

WHAT YOU'LL DO:

1. Preheat oven to 375°F.

2. Scrub and dry the potatoes. Place them on a rimmed baking sheet; bake in a 375°F oven for 30–40 minutes, or until the potatoes are tender. Remove the potatoes form the oven; let cool. When cooled, peel and discard the skins. Set aside.

3. Heat a large skillet over medium-high heat. Add oil; swirl to coat. Add onions; cook until tender and translucent, or about three minutes. Add garlic and cook 1 minute, stirring frequently. Add cumin, red and white ground peppers, salt, bone broth, and peptides. Bring to a boil, stirring occasionally.

4. Scoop half the bone broth mixture into a blender. Add two of the peeled, cooked sweet potatoes. Blend on high 2–3 minutes, or until smooth. Transfer to a large bowl. Repeat with the remaining broth mixture and potatoes.

5. Divide the soup evenly among 4 bowls. Sprinkle with cooked bacon, cheese, and chives, if desired.

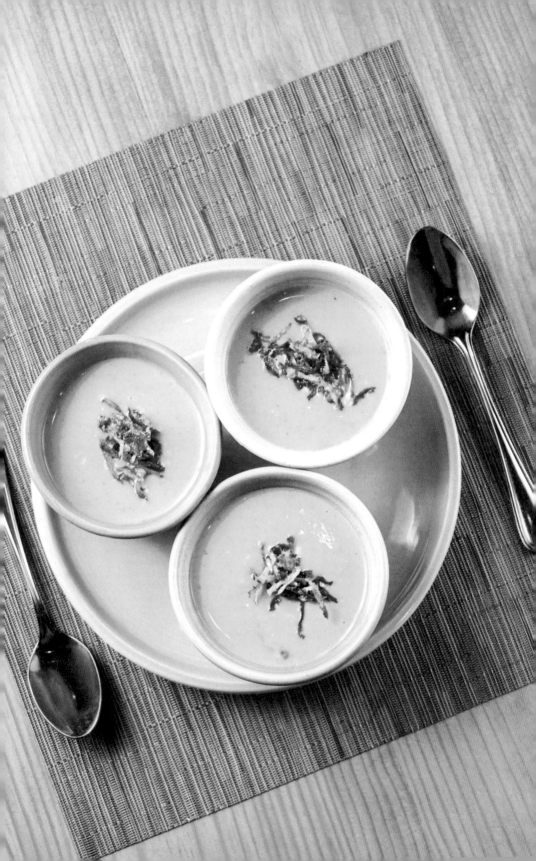

SPINACH-AND-CHICKEN-STUFFED SWEET POTATOES WITH CILANTRO-LIME SAUCE

Sweet potatoes are an incredible source of vitamin C, an antioxidant that boosts the immune system, fights free radicals, and jump-starts collagen synthesis. Getting enough vitamin C is vital to keeping collagen production running so you have enough for your bones, joints, skin, and more.

Makes 4 servings

STUFFED SWEET POTATOES

WHAT YOU'LL NEED:

- 4 medium sweet potatoes
- ½ cup chicken bone broth, homemade (page 78) or store-bought, or chicken stock
- ¼ teaspoon chili powder
- ½ teaspoon garlic powder
- ¼ teaspoon ground chipotle pepper
- ¼ teaspoon ground paprika

- 2 cups cooked, shredded rotisserie chicken
- 2 teaspoons olive oil
- 2 cloves garlic, minced
- 1¼ pounds baby spinach
- ¼ teaspoon kosher salt
- ¼ teaspoon freshly ground black pepper

CILANTRO-LIME SAUCE

WHAT YOU'LL NEED:

- ½ cup Greek yogurt
- 2 tablespoons finely chopped cilantro

- Juice from ½ lime
- ¼ teaspoon kosher salt

1. Preheat oven to 425°F. Wash and arrange the potatoes on an aluminum foil-lined rimmed baking sheet. Place on the oven's center rack; bake for 45 minutes, or until tender. Meanwhile, make the Cilantro-Lime Sauce.

2. In a small bowl, combine the yogurt, cilantro, lime juice, and salt. Cover and place in the refrigerator to chill.

3. Heat a small saucepan over medium heat. Combine the broth, chili and garlic powders, chipotle pepper, and paprika. Stir, and add the chicken. Warm the mixture on low to heat the chicken.

4. Heat a medium skillet over medium-high heat. Add oil to the pan; swirl to coat. Add the garlic and cook for 1 minute. Add the spinach. Stir occasionally until fully wilted, about 3 minutes.

5. When the potatoes are tender, make a lengthwise cut along each one to open, but do not cut through entirely. Using a towel, grip each end and gently push toward the center until the potato flesh is exposed. Evenly divide salt and pepper among the potatoes. Top with wilted spinach, chicken, and Cilantro-Lime Sauce.

CHICKEN FETTUCCINE WITH CREAMY COLLAGEN PASTA SAUCE

This isn't your typical creamy fettuccine alfredo, but you can use bone broth, coconut cream, and flour to make a palate-pleasing pasta sauce that's worth fighting over for the last spoonful.

Makes 4 servings

WHAT YOU'LL NEED:

- 8 ounces fettuccine
- 1 teaspoon olive oil
- 1 pound boneless, skinless chicken thighs, cut into bite-size pieces
- ¼ cup water
- 1 head broccoli, cut into pieces

PASTA SAUCE

WHAT YOU'LL NEED:

- 2 cloves garlic, minced
- 2 tablespoons whole-wheat flour
- 2 teaspoons lemon zest
- ½ cup coconut milk or whipping cream
- ½ cup chicken bone broth, homemade (page 78) or store-bought
- 4 scoops unflavored or chicken-flavored collagen peptides
- 1 tablespoon chopped fresh thyme
- 1 tablespoon chopped fresh oregano
- ½ teaspoon kosher salt
- ½ teaspoon freshly ground black pepper
- ¼ cup freshly grated Parmesan cheese

WHAT YOU'LL DO:

1. Cook pasta according to package directions. Strain and keep warm.

2. Heat a medium skillet over medium-high heat. Add oil to the pan; swirl to coat. Cook the chicken thighs for 6–7 minutes, stirring occasionally until cooked through and no longer pink when cut open with a knife. Remove the chicken from the pan.

3. Add the water and broccoli to the skillet. Cover and steam for 3–4 minutes, or until the broccoli pieces are tender. Remove the broccoli from the pan and set aside.

4. Without wiping out the skillet, sauté the garlic 1 minute. Add the flour, constantly stirring with a wooden spoon. Add the lemon zest, coconut milk, bone broth, and collagen peptides, and whisk until smooth, cooking for 3 minutes, or until the sauce begins to thicken. Add the thyme, oregano, salt, and pepper, and turn the heat to medium-low. Simmer for 10 minutes. Add the chicken, pasta, and broccoli to the skillet. Cook for 4 minutes, or until warmed through. Divide among four bowls. Top with Parmesan and serve.

TIP: If the sauce thickens too much, thin with 1 tablespoon bone broth; whisk until well incorporated.

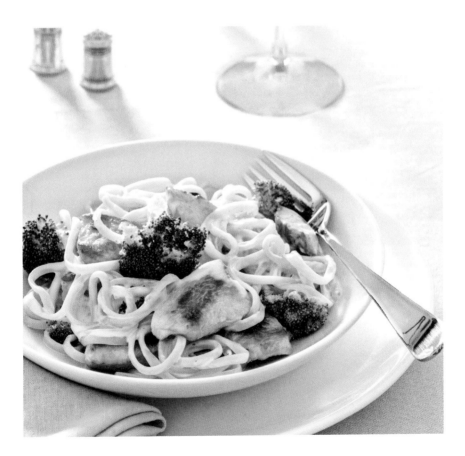

SHAKSHUKA

This Middle Eastern dish may have been designed originally for breakfast, but runny eggs over a spiced tomato mixture with sautéed veggies epitomizes the breakfast-for-dinner category.

Makes 4 servings

WHAT YOU'LL NEED:

- 2 tablespoons olive oil
- 1 cup chopped yellow onion
- 1 cup chopped red or orange bell pepper
- 3 cloves garlic, minced
- 2 scoops collagen peptides
- ¼ cup beef or chicken bone broth, homemade (page 78) or store-bought, or water
- 1 (28-ounce) can crushed tomatoes
- 1 teaspoon kosher salt

- 1 teaspoon chopped fresh oregano
- 1 tablespoon red wine vinegar
- 2 ounces feta cheese (about ½ cup), crumbled
- 4 large eggs
- ½ teaspoon freshly ground black pepper
- 2 tablespoons chopped fresh cilantro
- 4 ounces whole-wheat French baguette, sliced (approximately 24 slices)

WHAT YOU'LL DO:

1. Preheat oven to 375°F. Warm a large cast iron or oven-safe skillet over medium-high heat. Add oil to the pan; swirl to coat. Add the onion and bell pepper; sauté for 4–5 minutes, or until tender, stirring occasionally. Add the garlic and sauté for 2 more minutes, stirring occasionally. Add the collagen peptides and stir until incorporated.

2. Add the broth, tomatoes, salt, oregano, and vinegar to the mixture. Bring to a simmer and cook for 10–12 minutes, or until the sauce begins to thicken.

3. Sprinkle the feta over the tomato sauce. With the back of a large spoon, make four indentations in the tomato sauce. One at a time, crack each egg into a small bowl or cup and then gently pour it into one of the four indentations. Sprinkle the pepper over the eggs. Place the skillet in the oven and bake at 375°F for 12–15 minutes, or until the egg whites are set. Remove from the oven; sprinkle with cilantro and serve with bread.

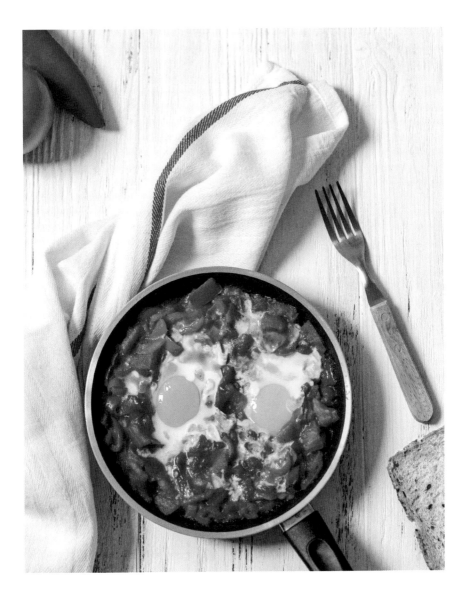

GRILLED SALMON WITH PUMPKIN SEED PESTO

Fish like salmon are a source of natural collagen as well as other vitamins and minerals essential to the collagen-producing process. If you pair salmon with collagen-boosting ingredients, you can make a big impact on your daily collagen goals.

Makes 4 servings

WHAT YOU'LL NEED:

- 1 pound salmon fillets, skin still intact
- 2 tablespoons olive oil
- ¼ teaspoon kosher salt
- ½ teaspoon freshly ground black pepper

WHAT YOU'LL DO:

1. Heat grill or grill pan to medium-high heat. Brush both sides of the fish fillets with oil. Evenly sprinkle salt and pepper over fillets. Grill skin-side down for 10 minutes, or until fish is flaky. Serve with Pumpkin Seed Pesto.

PUMPKIN SEED PESTO

If you have extra pesto, freeze it in ice cube trays. You can drop it into pan sauces or soups for a boost of flavor and nutrients.

Makes 6 servings

WHAT YOU'LL NEED:

- ½ cup pepitas (pumpkin seeds), shelled and roasted
- 2 cloves garlic
- 2 tablespoons grated pecorino Romano cheese
- 1 cup basil leaves
- ½ cup parsley leaves
- 4 tablespoons extra-virgin olive oil, divided
- 1 tablespoon fresh lemon juice
- ¼ teaspoon freshly ground black pepper

WHAT YOU'LL DO:

1. Add the pumpkin seeds, garlic, and cheese to a food processor. Pulse until the pumpkin seeds are almost ground and the garlic is finely chopped, about 20 seconds.

2. To the food processor bowl, add the basil, parsley, 2 tablespoons olive oil, lemon juice, and pepper. Pulse for about 30 seconds, scraping down the sides as needed. Add remaining 1 tablespoon oil if pesto mixture looks dry or clumpy. Stop pulsing when the pesto resembles a paste. Serve atop grilled salmon, or refrigerate for up to 2 days.

SALMON QUINOA BOWL WITH SESAME-LIME VINAIGRETTE

This crisp and refreshing quinoa bowl can serve as a weekday kitchen-sink meal of sorts. Keep the collagen-boosting basics—salmon, bell pepper, and cabbage—but mix and match with any grains, veggies, nuts or seeds you have on hand.

Makes 2 servings

SALMON QUINOA BOWL

WHAT YOU'LL NEED:

- 1 cup cooked quinoa
- ¼ cup julienned carrots
- ¼ chopped red bell pepper
- ¼ cup shredded red cabbage
- 6 ounces wild Alaskan salmon, broiled
- 2 tablespoons dry-roasted peanuts, chopped

SESAME-LIME VINAIGRETTE

WHAT YOU'LL NEED:

- 2 teaspoons soy sauce
- 2 tablespoons dark sesame oil
- 1 teaspoon lime juice
- 1 teaspoon rice vinegar

WHAT YOU'LL DO:

1. In a large bowl, combine the quinoa, carrots, bell pepper, and cabbage. Divide the mixture between two serving bowls. Top each bowl with salmon and sprinkle with peanuts.

2. In a small bowl, combine the soy sauce, dark sesame oil, lime juice, and rice vinegar, whisking well until combined. Divide and drizzle the mixture over each bowl.

WHY IS WILD SALMON BEST?

Wild salmon supplies a healthier ration of omega-3 fatty acids—the good kind you want for your brain and heart. Farm-raised salmon, on the other hand, often has higher proportions of omega-6 fatty acids, which are linked to inflammation. Plus, most wild-caught salmon today is sustainably harvested, which means their populations will be kept healthy for many more decades. Production conditions for farmed fish are often problematic, unless they are farmed in indoor recirculating tanks.

The majority of collagen in fish can be found in their bones, head, and fins, but smaller amounts are found in the meat. Supplement any fish or seafood you eat with collagen-boosting foods to get the most benefit from your plate.

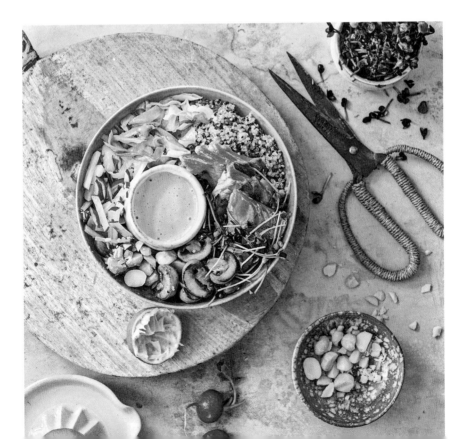

ALL-PURPOSE LEMON COLLAGEN VINAIGRETTE

Make a bottle of this homemade salad dressing on the weekend, then keep it nearby for a quick side salad or to drizzle over your weekly grilled chicken salad chock-full of veggies.

Makes 24 tablespoons

WHAT YOU'LL NEED:

- ¾ cup extra-virgin olive oil
- ¼ cup white wine vinegar
- 1 tablespoon lemon juice
- 1 teaspoon honey
- 2 scoops unflavored collagen peptides
- 2 tablespoons chopped fresh parsley
- 1 tablespoon chopped fresh oregano
- 1 shallot, peeled and minced
- ½ teaspoon kosher salt
- ½ teaspoon freshly ground black pepper

WHAT YOU'LL DO:

1. In a medium bowl, combine the oil, vinegar, lemon juice, honey, and peptides. Whisk until well combined and collagen peptides are dissolved. Add the remaining ingredients, whisking until just combined. Use the vinaigrette right away or store it in the fridge in a closed bottle for up to 1 week.

NOTE: If the vinaigrette has solidified when you remove it from the fridge, you can leave it at room temperature for 15 minutes to warm up. You can also run warm water over the outside of the bottle until the oil has returned to a liquid state.

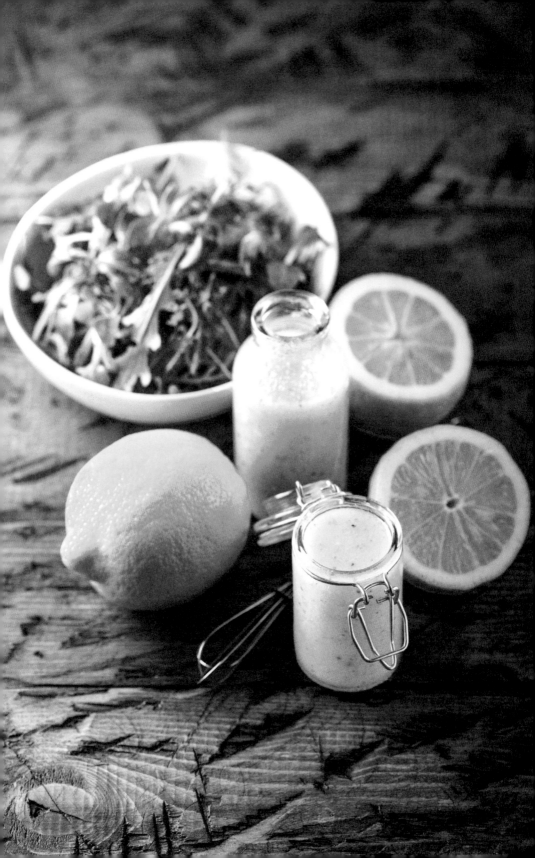

GREEN BEAN CASSEROLE

Green bean casserole is a staple of Thanksgiving and holiday dinners, but it's equally deserving of a spot on the weeknight dinner table. Let this speedy adaption—with collagen peptides, of course—help you get a heaping dose of comfort food any day of the week.

Makes 8 servings

WHAT YOU'LL NEED:

2½ pounds haricots verts, trimmed and cut into 2-inch pieces

1 tablespoon olive oil

1 medium yellow onion, thinly sliced

3 cups fresh button mushrooms, sliced

3 tablespoons whole-wheat flour

2 cups chicken bone broth, homemade (page 78) or store-bought

½ cup heavy cream

2 scoops unflavored collagen peptides

1 teaspoon kosher salt

¼ teaspoon freshly ground black pepper

½ cup whole-wheat panko breadcrumbs

⅓ cup grated Parmesan cheese

WHAT YOU'LL DO:

1. Blanch the haricots verts, then drain. Place in a 2-quart, broiler-safe baking dish.

2. Heat a large skillet over medium high. Add oil to the pan; swirl to coat. Add onion and mushrooms; cook until browned and water has evaporated, about 6–8 minutes.

3. Add flour and cook for 1 minute, stirring constantly. Add bone broth, heavy cream, peptides, salt, and pepper; whisk to fully incorporate. Cook for 4–6 minutes, stirring occasionally until sauce is smooth and thickened.

4. Spoon sauce over haricots verts. Top with breadcrumbs and Parmesan. Broil on high until golden brown, about 2 minutes.

SHAVED BRUSSELS SPROUTS SALAD WITH COLLAGEN-RICH DRESSING

Brussels sprouts don't have to be cooked to be tender and delicious enough to eat. Shaving them thin with a mandoline or julienning them into fine shreds makes the mini cabbage heads delicate enough to eat without the slightest bit of heat.

Makes 6 servings

SHAVED BRUSSELS SPROUTS SALAD

WHAT YOU'LL NEED:

- 1 pound Brussels sprouts, trimmed
- ½ cup toasted walnuts
- ½ cup dried cherries
- ¼ cup grated pecorino Romano cheese

COLLAGEN-RICH DRESSING

WHAT YOU'LL NEED:

- Zest and juice of 1 lemon
- 1 scoop unflavored collagen peptides
- 4 tablespoons extra-virgin olive oil or walnut oil
- 1 tablespoon white wine vinegar
- ¾ teaspoon kosher salt
- ½ teaspoon freshly ground black pepper

WHAT YOU'LL DO:

1. Thinly slice the Brussels sprouts on an adjustable mandoline or blade slicer. Place the Brussels sprouts into a medium mixing bowl. Add the walnuts, cherries, and cheese. Toss to combine, and set aside.

2. To make the dressing, in a small bowl, combine the lemon zest, peptides, oil, vinegar, salt, and pepper. Whisk well to combine. If the dressing is too thick, add water and stir, 1 teaspoon at a time. Spoon the dressing over the Shaved Brussels Sprouts Salad and toss to coat. Serve immediately.

SWEET POTATO NICE CREAM

Satisfy a craving for sweet potato pie in this ultra-creamy, incredibly decadent "Nice" Cream—a soft serve-style dessert that contains no dairy. It's also whipped up in a food processor instead of churned, so you can go from cravings to dessert in just a few moments (as long as you've prepped your ingredients ahead of time in anticipation of a future dessert need).

Makes 2 servings

WHAT YOU'LL NEED:

- 4 cubes pureed frozen sweet potato (about ½ cup) (see Tip)
- 2 frozen bananas, peeled and sliced
- 2 tablespoons sunflower or almond butter
- ½ teaspoon pure vanilla extract
- ½ teaspoon ground cinnamon
- 1 pinch ground nutmeg
- 1 scoop unflavored collagen peptides
- Unsweetened vanilla almond milk
- Sliced almonds, toasted coconut flakes, and bee pollen (optional)

WHAT YOU'LL DO:

1. Add the sweet potato cubes, banana, sunflower butter, vanilla extract, cinnamon, nutmeg, and peptides to a food processor. Process on medium speed for 2 minutes, or until texture resembles soft-serve ice cream, stopping to scrape down the sides of the bowl as needed. If the texture is too thick, add almond milk 1 tablespoon at a time. Scoop into two serving bowls and top with sliced almonds, coconut flakes, bee pollen, or other toppings of your preference. Serve immediately.

TIP: To make this Nice Cream come together quickly, cook the sweet potatoes, then scoop out the tender flesh, puree it, and freeze it in silicone ice cube trays. Standard trays hold 1 ounce in each well, or about 2 tablespoons. You'll need 4 cubes of frozen sweet potato puree for this sweet.

CHOCOLATE AVOCADO NICE CREAM

This Nice Cream hides a green secret. It might be chocolatey brown, but much of the creaminess comes from frozen avocado, which you may be able to find in your grocery store's frozen produce section. Avocado is rich in vitamin E, an antioxidant that helps prevent damage to collagen and works with vitamin C to synthesize more collagen in your body. For good measure (and even more chocolate flavor), add a scoop or two of a chocolate-flavored collagen supplement.

Makes 2 servings

WHAT YOU'LL NEED:

- 1 cup frozen avocado cubes
- 2 frozen bananas, peeled and sliced
- 1 tablespoon unsweetened cocoa powder or raw cacao (double if using unflavored collagen)
- 2 scoops chocolate-flavored or unflavored collagen peptides
- 1 tablespoon honey
- Unsweetened chocolate almond milk
- Cacao nibs, toasted chopped pecans, and toasted coconut flakes (optional)

WHAT YOU'LL DO:

1. Add the frozen avocado, banana, cocoa powder, peptides, and honey to a food processor. Process on medium speed for 2 minutes, or until texture resembles soft-serve ice cream, stopping to scrape down the sides of the bowl as needed. If the texture is too thick, add almond milk 1 tablespoon at a time. Scoop into two serving bowls; top with cacao nibs, pecans, coconut flakes, or other toppings of your choice. Serve immediately.

KEY LIME SQUARES WITH NUTTY GRAHAM CRACKER–COLLAGEN CRUST

Creamy lime squares are a refreshing treat after any meal. This dessert requires some effort, like your favorite key lime pie, but it's rich and decadent, so you only need a small square.

Makes 16 servings

CRUST

WHAT YOU'LL NEED:

- ⅔ cup shelled pistachios
- 18 graham crackers, crushed
- 2 scoops unflavored collagen peptides
- 1 tablespoon grated lime zest
- 5 tablespoons coconut oil

FILLING

WHAT YOU'LL NEED:

- 4 eggs
- ¾ cup key lime juice
- 1½ cups cane sugar
- ¼ cup rice flour
- 2 scoops unflavored collagen peptides

WHAT YOU'LL DO:

1. **For the crust:** Preheat oven to 350°F. Lightly grease and line a 9-inch square baking dish with parchment paper, leaving a 1- to 2-inch overhang on two sides of the pan.

2. In a food processor, grind the pistachios with the graham crackers, peptides, and lime zest. Stir in coconut oil until thoroughly combined. Pour the graham cracker mixture into the prepared dish. Using moistened hands, gently press into an even layer. Bake until light golden brown, about 10 minutes. Let cool completely.

3. **For the filling:** In a large bowl, combine the eggs with the lime juice. Add the sugar; whisk until smooth. Add the flour and peptides. Stir until just combined. Pour the filling into the cooled crust. Spread in an even layer.

4. Bake for 30–35 minutes, or until the filling is set and does not jiggle. Cool at room temperature for 1–2 hours. Using parchment paper overhangs, gently lift the bars out of the pan. Transfer to a cutting board and cut into squares.

TIP: Key limes are more aromatic, with greater floral notes compared to regular limes. They're also more tart. If you can't find key limes, you can substitute with a combination of regular lime juice and lemon juice in equal parts.

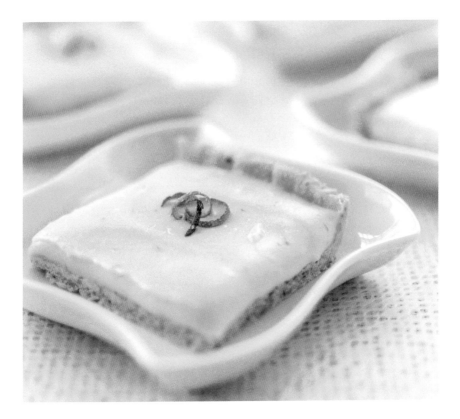

CHOCOLATE-TOPPED PUMPKIN-COLLAGEN FUDGE

You'll need a silicone ice cube tray for this recipe—a handy tool worth the few dollars it costs. You can use the same tray to freeze bone broth, pesto, or any other extra ingredients you want to make ahead of time and save for later.

Makes 6–8 servings (1 square per serving)

PUMPKIN FUDGE

WHAT YOU'LL NEED:

- ¼ cup almond butter
- 2 tablespoons pumpkin or sweet potato puree
- 2 teaspoons maple syrup
- 2 teaspoons coconut oil, melted
- 3 tablespoons almond flour
- 3 scoops unflavored or vanilla collagen peptides
- ¼ teaspoon ground cinnamon
- ⅛ teaspoon ground ginger
- ⅛ teaspoon ground nutmeg
- Pinch of ground cloves
- 1 tablespoon chopped dark chocolate

CHOCOLATE TOPPING

WHAT YOU'LL NEED:

- 2 tablespoons coconut oil
- 1 dark chocolate bar, at least 92% cocoa, chopped
- 2 teaspoons honey

1. **For Pumpkin Fudge:** Combine the almond butter, pumpkin puree, maple syrup, and coconut oil. Stir until well combined. In a small bowl, combine the flour, peptides, cinnamon, ginger, nutmeg, cloves, and chocolate. Fold this dry mixture into the pumpkin puree mixture. Gently divide the fudge among eight wells of a silicone ice cube tray, filling each well about halfway. Press each mixture down with the back of a spoon.

2. **For Chocolate Topping:** In a small saucepan, melt the coconut oil and chocolate bar, stirring occasionally. Add in the honey and stir to combine. Spoon chocolate evenly over each well of the pumpkin mixture.

3. Chill the chocolate-covered fudge in the freezer for 30 minutes, or until hard. Pop from molds and enjoy. Store remainders in the fridge in an airtight container for up to 4 days.

CHOCOLATE-COCONUT COLLAGEN BITES

Make a batch of these bites on the weekend, and keep them in an airtight container for your week's snacks. If you're going to be traveling, freeze a few before you leave, and package them in a jar or hard-sided container.

Makes 8 bites (1 bite per serving)

WHAT YOU'LL NEED:

- 1 cup coconut manna, softened
- 2 scoops unflavored or coconut-vanilla-flavored collagen peptides
- 1 tablespoon coconut oil
- 1 tablespoon cocoa powder
- 2 teaspoons honey
- ¾ cup shredded coconut, toasting optional, plus more for rolling
- 2 tablespoons rolled oats
- Finely chopped pecans, for rolling (optional)

WHAT YOU'LL DO:

1. In a large mixing bowl, combine the coconut manna, peptides, oil, cocoa powder, and honey, stirring well. Fold in the shredded coconut and rolled oats. Stir until just combined. If the mixture is too thick, add unsweetened coconut milk 1 teaspoon at a time.

2. Roll 1 tablespoon of the mixture into a ball. If desired, roll each ball through shredded coconut or finely chopped pecans for a light coating. Place in an airtight container and chill in the refrigerator for 1 hour, or until ready to eat. Keep the balls in the fridge for up to 5 days.

TIP: If your coconut manna is too solid and can't be scooped, you can soften it by dropping the jar in a bowl of hot water. Let it rest there for 5 minutes, then stir. Replace the hot water and let it soften a few minutes longer, or until you can stir the manna and scoop out enough for your recipe.

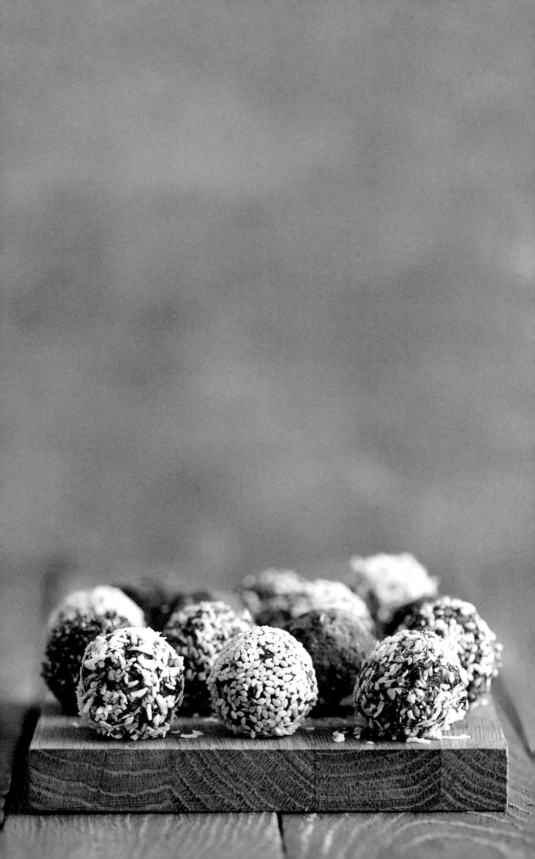

COOKIE DOUGH COLLAGEN BITES

Inspired by the cookie dough you once snuck from the fridge, these collagen-rich bites satisfy a sweet tooth with natural sweetening from dates and coconut.

Makes 12 bites (1 bite per serving)

WHAT YOU'LL NEED:

1 cup raw cashews

½ cup pitted dates, chopped

1 cup dried unsweetened coconut

¼ cup hemp seeds

1 teaspoon vanilla extract

2 scoops unflavored collagen peptides

3 tablespoons maple syrup

¼ cup dark chocolate, chopped

WHAT YOU'LL DO:

1. In a food processor, combine the cashews, dates, coconut, and hemp seeds. Pulse 1 minute. Add the vanilla extract, peptides, and maple syrup. Process for 1–2 minutes, or until a thick paste forms and the dough begins to ball up. Stop to scrape down the sides as needed. Remove the dough from the food processor and place it in a medium bowl. Add the dark chocolate to the bowl and fold with a spatula to combine.

2. Roll 2 teaspoons of dough into a ball. Store it in an airtight container in the refrigerator for up to 5 days.

ALMOND-CRANBERRY COLLAGEN SNACK BARS

Many snack bars deliver sugar and carbs, and few vitamins and minerals. Not only are these bars easy to make, they are a good source of collagen.

Makes 12 bars

WHAT YOU'LL NEED:

2 cups rolled oats

⅓ cup almond butter

¼ cup maple syrup

2 tablespoons coconut oil

3 scoops unflavored collagen peptides

1 teaspoon vanilla extract

½ teaspoon kosher salt

1 large egg white

⅓ cup dried cranberries, chopped

½ cup roasted almonds, coarsely chopped

WHAT YOU'LL DO:

1. Preheat oven to 350°F. Line an 8-inch square metal pan with parchment paper, leaving a 1- to 2-inch overhang on two sides of the pan.

2. Spread the oats on a rimmed baking sheet. Toast for 10–12 minutes in a 350°F oven, stirring at the halfway point. Once toasted, place in a medium mixing bowl and let cool completely.

3. In a small saucepan, combine the almond butter, maple syrup, and oil. Heat until the almond butter is melted; whisk to combine. Stir in the peptides, extract, salt, and egg white. Whisk to combine.

4. Add the cranberries and almonds to the cooled oats. Pour the almond butter mixture into the oats and stir until well combined. Spread the mixture into the parchment paper-lined metal pan. Use a spatula to firmly press the oat mixture down into the pan.

5. Bake at 350°F for 18–20 minutes, or until lightly browned. Let cool in the pan for 10 minutes. Using the parchment handles, lift the bars from the pan. Cool completely on a wire rack. Cut into 12 bars. Store it in an airtight container for up to 5 days.

TIP: To keep the bar mixture from sticking to your spatula as your press it into the pan, coat one side of the spatula with oil or cooking spray.

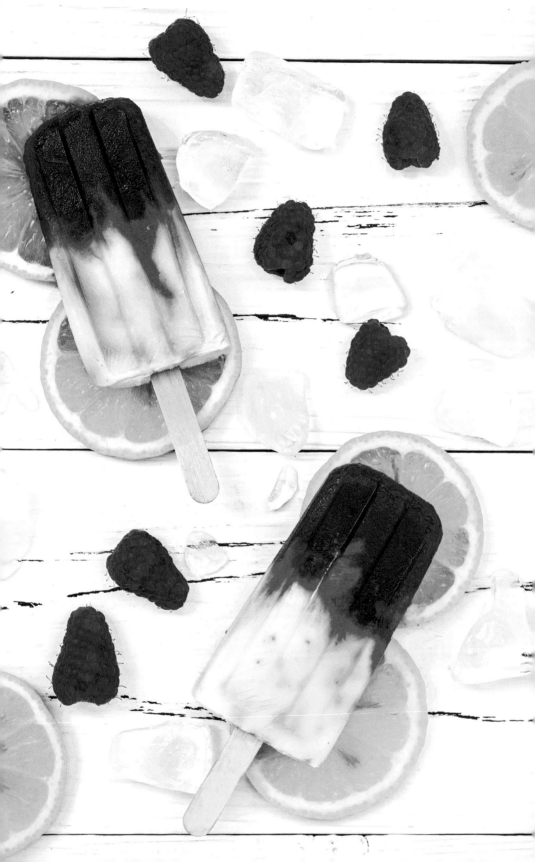

CREAMY COLLAGEN POPSICLES

Beat the heat with a collagen-boosting treat. This recipe uses blackberries, but you can substitute with any berries you have just so long as they provide the vitamin C your body needs to turn amino acids into strengthening collagen. You will need popsicle molds for this recipe.

Makes 6 servings

WHAT YOU'LL NEED:

- 2 tablespoons lemon juice
- 1 tablespoon honey
- 1 tablespoon water
- 1 cup fresh blackberries, or berry of your choice
- 1 cup organic coconut milk
- ¾ cup Greek vanilla yogurt
- 2 scoops unflavored collagen peptides

WHAT YOU'LL DO:

1. In a small saucepan, combine the lemon juice, honey, and water. Warm until just hot. Add the blackberries and stir to warm, about 3 minutes. Pour the berry mixture into a blender and blend on medium-high until smooth. Set aside.

2. In a medium bowl, combine the milk, yogurt, and collagen peptides. Whisk until smooth.

3. Pour each mixture into the molds, alternating layers of berry mixture with yogurt mixture until full. Use a long wooden skewer to gently swirl the layers in each mold. Place the handle portion of the mold, or a wooden tongue depressor, into the center of each pop. Freeze for at least 4–5 hours, or overnight, until hard.

BONE BROTH LATTE

While everyone else is sipping coffee or tea, you can sip on some skin-empowering collagen with a piping-hot cup of bone broth. For an extra-special treat every once in a while, turn that broth into a creamy, luxurious latte with the addition of coconut oil, an extra scoop of collagen peptides, and a hint of spice.

Makes 1 serving

WHAT YOU'LL NEED:

- 8 ounces beef bone broth, homemade (page 78) or store-bought
- Dash of ground ginger (optional)
- Dash of ground turmeric (optional)
- 1 tablespoon coconut oil
- 1 tablespoon organic grass-fed ghee
- 2 scoops unflavored collagen peptides
- Kosher salt, to taste

WHAT YOU'LL DO:

1. Bring the bone broth to a simmer over medium heat in a small saucepan. Whisk in the ginger and turmeric, if desired. Simmer for 1–2 minutes.

2. Transfer the bone broth mixture to a blender. Add the oil, ghee, and peptides. Blend on medium speed for 1 minute, or until frothy. Taste, and add salt to taste, blending as needed. Pour mixture into a large mug and enjoy.

ULTIMATE COLLAGEN LATTE

If your morning isn't complete without a jolt of caffeine, then have no fear: you can still get your buzz while boosting your daily collagen intake. This creamy latte combines your favorite coffee with collagen peptides and coconut oil for a filling and wonderfully rich beverage.

Makes 1 serving

WHAT YOU'LL NEED:

- 8 ounces freshly brewed hot coffee
- 2 tablespoons coconut oil
- 1–2 scoops unflavored collagen peptides
- 1 teaspoon pure vanilla extract
- Ground cinnamon or nutmeg (optional)

WHAT YOU'LL DO:

1. Place the coffee, oil, peptides, and vanilla extract into a blender. Blend for 60 seconds on medium speed, until frothy. Pour mixture into a large mug. Sprinkle it with cinnamon or nutmeg, if desired.

MATCHA COLLAGEN LATTE

Matcha powder is made from finely ground green tea leaves. It imparts a blissfully green color in any drink or dish and delivers a good dose of minerals and vitamins.

Makes 1 serving

WHAT YOU'LL NEED:

- 1 cup unsweetened vanilla almond milk or other milk as preferred
- ½ teaspoon matcha powder
- 2 teaspoons honey
- 1 scoop unflavored collagen peptides

WHAT YOU'LL DO:

1. Heat the almond milk in a small saucepan over medium heat. When simmering, pour the milk in the blender. Add the remaining ingredients and blend on low speed until frothy, 1–2 minutes. Pour into a large mug and enjoy.

TIP: If you have a blender that warms as it blends (for example, some Vitamix models), then you can skip the stovetop heating step. The blender will warm the milk while it froths all the ingredients.

CHOCOLATE COLLAGEN SMOOTHIE

Chill out and cool down with a fruit-filled smoothie that delivers vitamins, minerals, and a good dose of collagen peptides. This recipe calls for unflavored collagen peptides, but several brands make flavored options, including coconut or chocolate. You could substitute with one of those.

Makes 1 serving

WHAT YOU'LL NEED:

- 1 cup unsweetened vanilla oat milk or other milk as preferred
- 1 frozen sliced banana
- 2 tablespoons almond or peanut butter
- 3 tablespoons raw cacao powder
- 1 scoop unflavored collagen peptides or flavor of your choice
- ½ tablespoon honey (optional)

WHAT YOU'LL DO:

1. Add all ingredients to the blender, including the honey, if desired. Blend on medium speed for 30 seconds. Increase speed to high and blend until the mixture is thick and smooth.

HAVE FRUIT THAT'S ALMOST OVERRIPE? Cut it into slices or chunks, freeze it, and save it for your next smoothie.

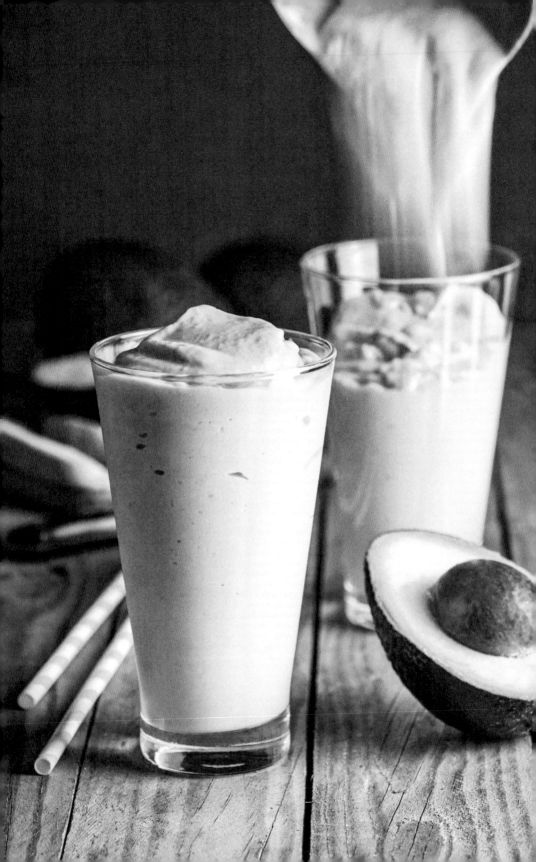

GREAT GREEN COLLAGEN SMOOTHIE

Avocado and matcha powder are rich sources of antioxidants, polyphenols, and other disease-fighting nutrients. Avocado also happens to be a good source of heart-healthy monounsaturated fats. Packing these healthful ingredients into a sippable, collagen-boosting smoothie is an easy way to treat your body to a great host of benefits as you're drinking something incredibly delicious and refreshing.

Makes 1 serving

WHAT YOU'LL NEED:

- 1 cup unsweetened almond milk or other milk as preferred
- 1 frozen sliced banana
- ½ cup frozen cubed mango
- ½ avocado, cubed and frozen (about ½ cup)
- 1–2 teaspoons matcha powder
- 1 scoop unflavored or coconut-flavored collagen peptides

WHAT YOU'LL DO:

1. Add all ingredients to the blender. Blend on medium speed for 30 seconds. Increase speed to high and blend until mixture is thick and smooth.

PREP TIP: MAKE SMOOTHIE FREEZER PACKS

Speed up your smoothie process by making freezer packs of smoothie ingredients. When you're ready to blend up a cup brimming with healthful ingredients, you can skip the step of hauling out boxes, jars, and jugs and instead reach for your premade and premeasured pack of ingredients instead.

Consider what combination of fruits or vegetables you would like, then prep accordingly, chopping your chosen ingredients into 2- to 3-inch chunks. To a zip-top bag, add all prepared fruits and vegetables (this includes any greens). With a permanent marker or wax pen, label the bag with the ingredients or smoothie name and put it in the freezer.

When you're ready to blend, add the liquids, such as nondairy milk, to the blender first. Dump in the smoothie pack ingredients. Add collagen peptides, sweeteners, and other nonfrozen ingredients, including nut butters. Blend until smooth, then enjoy.

MINT-CHIP COLLAGEN SMOOTHIE

For fans of mint-chocolate chip ice cream—or any combination of fresh mint and creamy chocolate, really—this smoothie is the treat you deserve.

Makes 1 serving

WHAT YOU'LL NEED:

- ¾ cup unsweetened almond milk or other milk as preferred
- 1 cup spinach
- 3 tablespoons fresh mint leaves, torn
- 1 frozen sliced banana

- 1 tablespoon cacao nibs (or 2 tablespoons, if using unflavored collagen)
- 1 scoop unflavored or chocolate-flavored collagen peptides
- ½ tablespoon honey (optional)

WHAT YOU'LL DO:

1. Add all ingredients to the blender, including honey, if desired. Blend on medium speed for 30 seconds. Increase speed to high and blend until mixture is thick and smooth.

WATERMELON COLLAGEN SLUSH

When the sun is strong and the thirst is real, cool down with a fruit slush that's reminiscent of childhood. This one, however, is more than sugary syrup, artificial coloring, and ice. Frozen fruit makes a great base for these icy concoctions. If you don't have frozen fruit, fresh will do—just add more ice.

Makes 2 servings

WHAT YOU'LL NEED:

1½ cups cubed and deseeded frozen watermelon

1 cup frozen halved strawberries

2 tablespoons lime juice

1–2 scoops unflavored or berry-flavored collagen peptides

Ice

WHAT YOU'LL DO:

1. Add all ingredients to a blender with 1 cup ice. Blend on medium speed for 30 seconds. Increase speed to high and blend until mixture is thick and smooth. If the slush is too thin, add more ice. If it's too thick, add more lime juice or water.

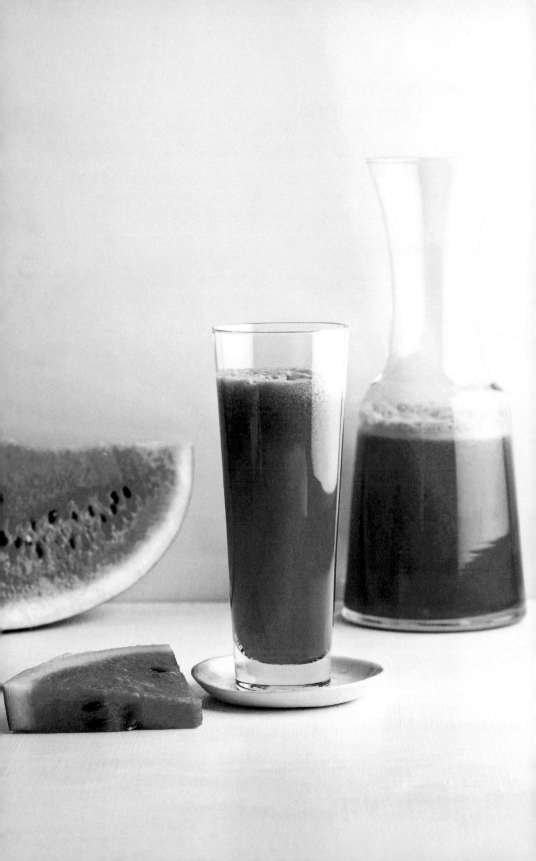

LEMON-MINT COLLAGEN-INFUSED WATER

Bottled collagen waters are making their way onto grocery store shelves, but why buy when you can DIY? Fresh fruit, water, and collagen peptides are all you need to make this refreshing drink. If using sill water, make this up to 2 days in advance to let the fruit juices fully infuse the water.

Makes 4–8 servings

WHAT YOU'LL NEED:

- 1 lemon, sliced
- ½ cup mint leaves, torn
  Filtered still water or sparkling water
- 2 scoops unflavored collagen peptides (or the flavor of your choice)

WHAT YOU'LL DO:

1. To a juice jar or pitcher, add the lemon slices and mint leaves. Top with enough water to fill the container and add collagen, stirring until combined. Chill, and then serve over ice.

BOTTOMS UP! When you've drained the water, you can snack on the fruit for fiber, vitamins, and minerals.

TASTY INFUSED WATER COMBINATIONS

Staying hydrated keeps skin cells plump, which can reduce fine lines and wrinkles. This collagen-enhanced water just happens to have the added benefit of doing even more work for your skin, joins, and bones.

CITRUS-BLUEBERRY-BASIL

1 cup blueberries

1 orange, sliced

1 cup basil leaves, torn

Filtered still water or sparklingwater

2 scoops unflavored collagen peptides (flavor of choice)

RASPBERRY-LIME-MINT

1 cup raspberries, muddled

1 lime, sliced

1 cup mint leaves, torn

Filtered still water or sparkling water

2 scoops unflavored collagen peptides (flavor of choice)

PEACH-ROSEMARY

2 peaches, sliced

½ lemon, sliced

6 sprigs rosemary

Filtered still water or sparkling water

2 scoops unflavored collagen peptides (flavor of choice)

STRAWBERRY-GINGER-THYME

1 cup strawberries, sliced

¼ cup ginger, peeled and sliced

6 sprigs thyme

Filtered still water or sparkling water

2 scoops unflavored collagen peptides (flavor of choice)

WATERMELON-CUCUMBER-MINT

2 cups cubed watermelon

½ cucumber, sliced

1 cup mint leaves, torn

Filtered still water or sparkling water

2 scoops unflavored collagen (flavor of choice)

ORANGE DREAM DRINK

My, what a sweet sip! This orange drink blends collagen peptides with vitamin C, a necessary antioxidant in the collagen synthesis process.

Makes 1 serving

WHAT YOU'LL NEED:

- 1 cup orange juice
- 2 tablespoons coconut milk
- 1 scoop unflavored collagen peptides
- ½ teaspoon honey
- 1 cup ice
- 1 orange slice (for garnish)

WHAT YOU'LL DO:

1. Add all ingredients to the blender and process until smooth. Add more ice if you like a thicker texture. Garnish with an orange slice, if desired.

WHICH IS BETTER: FLAVORED OR UNFLAVORED COLLAGEN PEPTIDES?

A variety of flavored collagen peptides is available today, from coconut and berry to chocolate or matcha beef. What you buy should depend largely on how you plan to ingest it. If your primary collagen intake will come from smoothies, drinks, and soups, you might consider an unflavored option. It's versatile, and you won't risk it sitting unused and waiting for special recipes only.

However, if you have a variety of recipe plans for the collagen you're purchasing, consider picking up a few different flavors. Beef, chicken, and marine collagen are likely best for savory options. Sweeter dishes can benefit from some flavored options with fruity or tropical undertones.

SWEETENED COLLAGEN ICED TEA

Seriously yummy and delicately sweet, this chilled collagen tea is a great make-ahead beverage option for picnics, backyard barbecues, or just those days when you want a little bit more oomph in your drink.

Makes 4 servings

WHAT YOU'LL NEED:

- 6 cups water
- 4 chamomile tea bags
- 4 lemon herbal tea bags
- ¼ cup coconut milk

- 4 teaspoons honey
- 2 scoops unflavored collagen peptides
- 1 lemon cut into wedges (for garnish)

WHAT YOU'LL DO:

1. In a medium saucepan, bring the water to a boil. Add both varieties of tea bags and let them steep for 4 minutes, or until the preferred concentration is achieved. Stir in the coconut milk, honey, and peptides.

2. Pour the mixture into an iced tea pitcher and cool it in the refrigerator for at least 1 hour. Serve over ice with a lemon wedge and enjoy!

TIP: If you prefer your tea piping hot, serve this sweetened tea immediately after combining all the ingredients. It's equally delicious warm.

GUMMIES

Gummies may remind you of childhood fruit snacks, but adults get to revisit their younger days with these chewy, snappy treats. Gummies are ideal snacks for collagen seekers because peptides blend so beautifully into the final product. Keep a set of silicone molds on hand—that way you'll always have a fresh batch of gummies ready when a craving strikes. Silicone ice molds are fine, but for fancier shapes, seek out chocolate molds. They come in a variety of fun options, from seashells to holiday wreaths.

HONEY-TURMERIC COLLAGEN GUMMIES

Honey and turmeric are a favorite combo for warm tea, but they also make a wonderfully spiced gummy.

Makes about 12 servings

WHAT YOU'LL NEED:

- 3½ scoops of unflavored collagen peptides
- ½ cup cold water
- 1 cup coconut milk
- 1 tablespoon ground turmeric
- Dash of ground cinnamon
- 1 tablespoon honey

WHAT YOU'LL DO:

1. Place the collagen peptides into a small mixing bowl. Slowly stir the cold water into the peptides, mixing with a whisk. When fully combined, let it sit for 5 minutes, or until the combination is rubbery.

2. In a small saucepan over low heat, combine the coconut milk, turmeric, cinnamon, and honey. Slowly whisk in the collagen mixture. Stir until the collagen and spices are completely dissolved without lumps. Do not let the mixture boil.

3. Pour the mixture into silicone molds. Place the molds in the refrigerator until firm, about 45 minutes. Once hardened and firm, remove the gummies from the molds. Store them in an airtight container in the refrigerator for up to 5 days.

BLACKBERRY-LEMON KOMBUCHA GUMMIES

Gelatin, a product of collagen, is typically only used in hot dishes because cold temperatures turn it from a liquid to a gel. However, you can use this quality to your advantage by turning the thick gelatin into a sweet gummy.

Makes about 20 servings

WHAT YOU'LL NEED:

1 cup kombucha

3 scoops beef gelatin (about 6 tablespoons)

2 cups blackberries

2 tablespoons lemon juice

3 tablespoons honey

WHAT YOU'LL DO:

1. In a medium bowl, combine the kombucha and gelatin. Set aside and let the gelatin bloom, about 5 minutes.

2. In a blender, combine the blackberries, lemon juice, and honey. Blend on high speed until smooth. Strain the mixture into another bowl through a cheesecloth. Discard solids.

3. Pour the remaining blackberry mixture into a medium saucepan and warm over low heat until hot but not simmering. Remove from the heat and add the bloomed gelatin. Whisk until well combined.

4. Spoon the mixture into silicone molds or an 8 × 8–inch glass baking dish lightly coated with oil. Place in the refrigerator until firm, about 1 hour. If using a baking dish, slice with a serrated knife to form 20 squares; if using silicone molds, remove the gummies from the mold. Store in an airtight container for up to 2 weeks. Place sheets of wax paper between any layers to keep gummies from sticking.

CRANBERRY-CITRUS COLLAGEN GUMMIES

These gummies can be fun around the holidays, when cranberries and zippy citrus are in everything from sparkling waters to cocktails. But the ingredients are evergreen, so there's no harm in making these for a day by the pool.

Makes about 20 servings

WHAT YOU'LL NEED:

- ½ cup fresh orange juice, strained
- 3 scoops beef gelatin (about 6 tablespoons)
- ¾ cup cranberry juice
- 1 tablespoon honey

WHAT YOU'LL DO:

1. In a small bowl, combine the orange juice and gelatin. Stir to combine.

2. Let it sit to bloom, about 5 minutes.

3. In a small saucepan, heat the cranberry juice and honey until hot but not simmering. Stir occasionally. Remove from heat. Slowly add in the bloomed gelatin mixture, whisking constantly. Continue to stir until the gelatin is fully dissolved, about 8 minutes.

4. Once all the lumps are out of the liquid, pour the juice mixture into silicone molds or a 8 × 8–inch glass baking dish lightly coated with oil. Refrigerate for 1–2 hours, or until firm. If using a baking dish, slice into 20 squares using a serrated knife. Store them in an airtight container for up to 2 weeks.

SUMMER MELON COLLAGEN GUMMIES

When the farmers' market tables are weighted down with melons, it's time to grab a few to make these refreshing gummies.

Makes about 20 servings

WHAT YOU'LL NEED:

¼ cup water or juice of choice

3 tablespoons honey

3 cups cubed ripe melon, such as honeydew or cantaloupe

4 tablespoons beef gelatin

WHAT YOU'LL DO:

1. In a medium saucepan, combine the water and honey. Warm over low-medium heat, stirring to dissolve the honey. When the honey is dissolved, add the melon. Heat until the melon is warm, about 8 minutes.

2. Spoon the mixture into a blender. Blend on medium speed for 1–2 minutes, or until smooth. Add the gelatin and let it sit to bloom, 3–5 minutes. Blend on low speed to thoroughly combine.

3. Spoon the mixture into silicone molds or a lightly greased 8 × 8–inch baking dish. Chill in the refrigerator for 1–2 hours, or until firm. Store the gummies in an airtight container for up to 2 weeks. Place sheets of wax paper between multiple layers of gummies, if needed, to keep them from sticking.

A 3-DAY COLLAGEN MENU

Get started on a collagen-rich diet with
these three days of suggested menus.

DAY 1

* **Breakfast:** Greek yogurt with strawberries and walnuts, plus one scoop of collagen peptides
* **Lunch:** Sweet Potato-Greens Hash (page 70)
* **Dinner:** Bone Broth Ramen (page 87)
* **Snacks:** Almonds and a hard-boiled egg

DAY 2

* **Breakfast:** Great Green Collagen Smoothie (page 123)
* **Lunch:** Spinach- and Chicken-Stuffed Sweet Potatoes with Cilantro-Lime Sauce (page 92)
* **Dinner:** Shakshuka (page 96)
* **Snacks:** Blueberries and toasted pepitas

DAY 3

* **Breakfast:** Oatmeal Banana Pancakes (page 77)
* **Lunch:** Chicken Zoodle Soup (page 84)
* **Dinner:** Salmon Quinoa Bowl with Sesame-Lime Vinaigrette (page 100)
* **Snacks:** Clementine and carrots with hummus

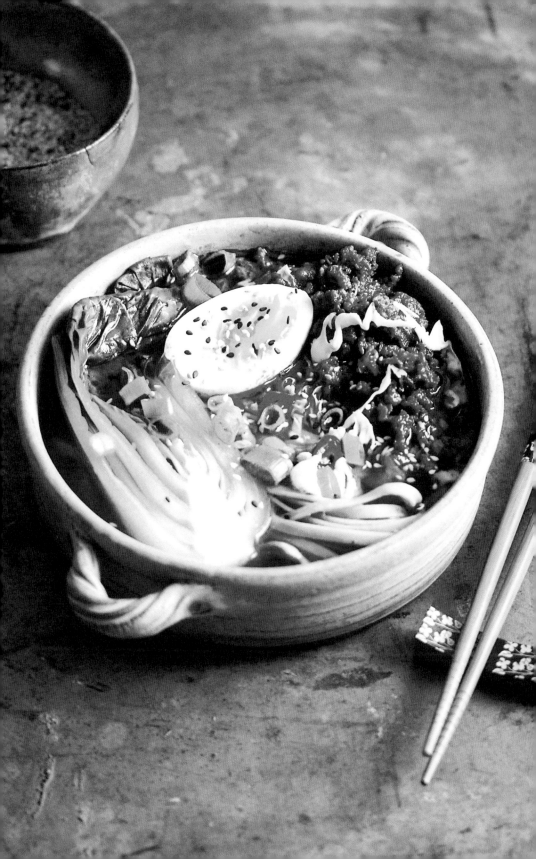

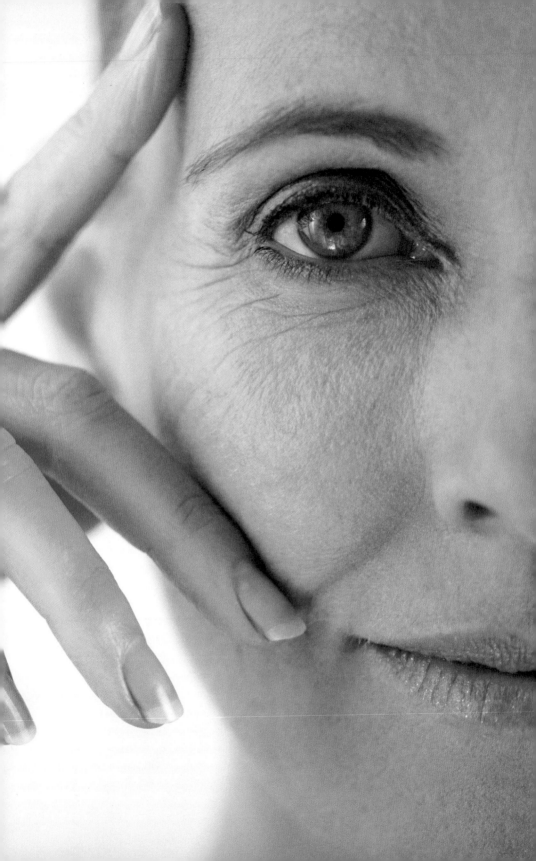

PART 4

Frequently Asked Questions

What is collagen?

Collagen is the most abundant type of protein in the human body. It combines with other natural materials, like minerals and vitamins, to form many parts of the human body, from bones and teeth to skin, organs, and muscles. Your body makes some collagen, but with age, it produces less and less. You can supplement collagen—and reap many potential health benefits—by eating a diet filled with collagen-rich foods and collagen-boosting ones, too. Supplements, including collagen peptides, can help stimulate your body's natural synthesis and boost your collagen quantity.

Where is collagen?

Collagen is in everything. It makes up the majority of the white part of your eyes, and it's the primary component in connective tissues like tendons and cartilage. Skin layers are filled with collagen, and, when combined with elastin, it's responsible for the skin's supple, hydrated, and youthful appearance. Collagen is also used to make bones, and a small percentage of muscle is made from collagen.

Does your body make its own collagen?

It does until you're about thirty years old. For the first three decades of your life, collagen production and replacement keep pace, but around age thirty, collagen production begins falling off. That's when visible signs of aging begin to appear, including thinning skin, wrinkles, and fine lines.

How much collagen is helpful? How much is safe to consume in one day?

The average person will see benefits with a dose between 2.5 and 12 grams. However, studies have looked at doses as high as 15 grams and not found any negative impacts. There is no established daily amount, so you can begin with 2.5 grams in a day and build your way up as long as you don't experience side effects like gastric bloating or upset stomach.

What health benefits do you get from collagen?

Collagen is still being studied, so new possible benefits seem to pop up every year. However, the majority of the research that exists now points toward collagen being most helpful with:

* Building and strengthening bones
* Protecting joints by revitalizing cartilage
* Improving signs of aging on skin
* Protecting the heart
* Building muscles and slowing deterioration

Are there any risks to taking collagen supplements?

So far, research has identified no serious side effects associated with taking collagen supplements. Because collagen occurs naturally in foods, most people can tolerate supplements well. If you are allergic to the source of the collagen (fish, for example), then you won't be able to use those supplements. If you develop side effects like upset stomach, nausea, gastric discomfort, or bloating, try taking less of the supplement to see if a large dose is just too difficult for your body to process at first.

What studies have been conducted on the health benefits of collagen supplements?

Research into collagen is relatively new, though scientists have known about the protein for decades. The most significant area of research relates to collagen's effects on skin. Other topics, such as bone health and heart health, are still relatively new, but the studies that have been released are promising.

It's important to understand that many collagen tests are first conducted on animals, such as rats or mice, before they're conducted on humans. Wherever possible, human tests were preferred and used as the support for the assertions in this book. If an animal or cell study were the only studies available, this was noted.

Is it better to eat collagen-rich foods or take collagen supplements?
Both. Researchers don't know how well the body absorbs collagen from either source, though it's clear they both have a beneficial impact, as studies have found significant improvements. You can continue to seek out the protein from collagen-rich foods while supplementing with collagen peptides as needed or regularly, such as through a daily supplement.

Does cooking destroy the collagen in collagen supplements?
No. Gelatin and collagen go through several heat stages, so a little extra heat in the cooking process won't destroy the helpful proteins.

How many calories are in a tablespoon of collagen? Two scoops?
A tablespoon of collagen peptides that do not have any added sweeteners equals about 35 calories. Most collagen manufacturers include a two-tablespoon scoop in every jar, so one scoop would be about 70 calories.

What nutrients are commonly found in collagen supplements?
Collagen is a protein, so scoops of collagen are a good source of protein. The average two-tablespoon scoop has about 9 grams of protein, which is more protein than what's in an egg.

Plus, of course, collagen contains collagen—about 10 grams in one scoop. Some unflavored collagen peptides also contain sodium. That can range from 40 to 60 milligrams per scoop.

Is there anything you should avoid in a collagen supplement?
It's best if you look for (and support by purchasing) collagen supplements that are made from grass-fed, pasture-raised animals or wild-caught fish

and seafood. These animal sources are not given antibiotics or chemicals that could render a lower-quality collagen product. Plus, collagen sources from many conventionally raised animals don't produce the type of high-quality collagen that's necessary for the full benefits.

Also, use collagen supplements without any artificial sweeteners. As the market of high-quality collagen supplements has begun to embrace flavors (vanilla coconut, matcha, berry, and more), you might find some that use these fake sugars and some that don't. Just be sure to read the labels and look for ones that are preservative-free.

METRIC CONVERSION CHART

US SYSTEM	METRIC SYSTEM
Volume	
1 teaspoon	5 milliliters
1 tablespoon	15 milliliters
¼ cup	60 milliliters
½ cup	120 milliliters
¾ cup	180 milliliters
1 cup	240 milliliters
1 quart	960 milliliters
Weight	
4 ounces	113 grams
8 ounces	227 grams
12 ounces	340 grams
16 ounces	454 grams
Temperature	
300°F	150°C
325°F	160°C
350°F	180°C
375°F	190°C
400°F	200°C
425°F	220°C
450°F	230°C
Baking Pan Size	
8x8x2 inches	20x20x5 centimeters

GLOSSARY

Amino acids: Protein building blocks that combine to form long strands of collagen—and, eventually, triple helices—that become collagen fibrils and fibers.

Antioxidants: Compounds that can help prevent damage to layers of skin, stop collagen destruction, and possibly help amino acids generate more proteins.

Collagen: The most significant structural protein in the human body.

Collagen fibrils: Long strands of collagen that bunch together side by side for immense strength and durability.

Collagen hydrolysate: Also known as *hydrolyzed collagen*; collagen that has been processed, broken down into shorter amino acid chains, and turned into a form that can be used as a supplement, such as a powder.

Extracellular matrix: Also called the ECM; a network of collagen, molecules, cells, and other materials that (1) forms the "skeleton" of many tissues, including bones and muscles, and (2) holds together the many tissues and organs inside the body.

Gelatin: A fatty substance rendered from collagen-rich products; often dehydrated and sold in capsules, powders, or sheets so that it can be rehydrated and added back to food for health benefits.

Helix: A three-strand collection of tightly bound collagen strands that produce some of collagen's characteristics, including elasticity and strength.

Peptides: Another name for *hydrolyzed collagen*, or collagen that has been processed for easier absorption when taken as a supplement.

Placebo: A substance or product given to test subjects that has no active properties; placebos help researchers determine if any changes in the group given the active ingredient are a result of the ingredient or of another measure.

Procollagen: A pre-collagen form of the protein that is still strong and durable but needs to go through another stage of synthesis in order to become collagen.

RESOURCES

Brands We Recommend

* Ancient Nutrition – ancientnutrition.com

* Bonafide Provisions – bonafideprovisions.com

* Brodo – brodo.com

* Bulletproof – bulletproof.com

* Primal Kitchen – primalkitchen.com

* Vital Proteins – vitalproteins.com

BIBLIOGRAPHY

"Albert Szent-Györgyi." The Nobel Prize. Accessed May 10, 2019. https://www.nobelprize.org/prizes/medicine/1937/szent-gyorgyi/biographical/.

"Articular Cartilage Restoration." OrthoInfo. Accessed April 3, 2019. https://orthoinfo.aaos.org/en/treatment/articular-cartilage-restoration/.

"Best Way You Can Get More Collagen." Cleveland Clinic. Accessed February 15, 2019. https://health.clevelandclinic.org/the-best-way-you-can-get-more-collagen/.

"Collagen May Help Protect Brain Against Alzheimer's Disease." ScienceDaily. Accessed May 3, 2019. https://www.sciencedaily.com/releases/2008/12/081210150713.htm.

"Epithelial Cells." Arizona State University. Accessed March 5, 2019. https://askabiologist.asu.edu/epithelial-cells.

"Epithelial Cells in Urine." MedlinePlus. Accessed March 5, 2019. https://medlineplus.gov/lab-tests/epithelial-cells-in-urine/.

"IUPUI Professor Lands NIH Grant to Research Methods to Strengthen Bones, Resist Fractures." Indiana University. Accessed March 2, 2019. https://news.iu.edu/stories/2018/09/iupui/releases/04-nih-grant-research-bone-fractures-osteoporosis-collagen.html.

"Osteoporosis." National Institute on Aging. Accessed April 5, 2019. https://www.nia.nih.gov/health/osteoporosis.

"Osteoporosis Overview." NIH Osteoporosis and Related Bone Diseases National Resource Center. Accessed April 5, 2019. https://www.bones.nih.gov/health-info/bone/osteoporosis/overview.

"Salmon Overview." Monterey Bay Aquarium Seafood Watch. Accessed May 10, 2019. https://www.seafoodwatch.org/seafood-recommendations/groups/salmon/overview?q=Salmon&t=salmon.

"U.S. Leading Categories of Diseases/Disorders." National Institute of Mental Health. Accessed April 11, 2019. https://www.nimh.nih.gov/health/statistics/disability/us-leading-categories-of-diseases-disorders.shtml.

"Vitamin A." National Institutes of Health. Accessed May 3, 2019. https://ods.od.nih.gov/factsheets/VitaminA-HealthProfessional/.

"Vitamin C." National Institutes of Health. Accessed May 3, 2019. https://ods.od.nih.gov/factsheets/VitaminC-HealthProfessional/.

"What Is a Standard Drink?" National Institute on Alcohol Abuse and Alcoholism. Accessed May 10, 2019. https://www.niaaa.nih.gov/alcohol-health/overview-alcohol-consumption/what-standard-drink.

"What Is Osteoarthritis?" Arthritis Foundation. Accessed April 5, 2019. https://www.arthritis.org/about-arthritis/types/osteoarthritis/what-is-osteoarthritis.php.

"What Is Photoaging?" Skin Cancer Foundation. Accessed May 6, 2019. https://www.skincancer.org/healthy-lifestyle/anti-aging/what-is-photoaging.

Adam, M., et al. "Postmenopausal osteoporosis. Treatment with calcitonin and a diet rich in collagen proteins." *Casopis Lékaru Ceských* 135, no. 3 (1996): 74–8. Accessed April 9, 2019. https://www.ncbi.nlm.nih.gov/pubmed/8625373.

Alvares, Thiago Silveira, et al. "Acute L-Arginine Supplementation Does Not Increase Nitric Oxide Production in Healthy Subjects." *Nutrition & Metabolism* 9 (2012): 54. Accessed May 6, 2019. https://www.ncbi.nlm.nih.gov/pmc/articles/PMC3489573/.

Asserin, J., et al. "The Effect of Oral Collagen Peptide Supplementation on Skin Moisture and the Dermal Collagen Network: Evidence from an Ex Vivo Model and Randomized, Placebo-Controlled Clinical Trials." *Journal of Cosmetic Dermatology* 14, no. 4 (2015): 291–301. Accessed March 1, 2019. https://www.ncbi.nlm.nih.gov/pubmed/26362110.

Avila Rodriguez, M. I., et al. "Collagen: A Review on Its Sources and Potential Cosmetic Applications." *Journal of Cosmetic Dermatology* 17, no. 1 (2018): 20–6. Accessed February 15, 2019. https://www.ncbi.nlm.nih.gov/pubmed/29144022.

Bello, A. E., et al. "Collagen Hydrolysate for the Treatment of Osteoarthritis and Other Joint Disorders: A Review of the Literature." *Current Medical Research and Opinion* 22, no. 11 (2006): 2221–32. Accessed March 3, 2019. https://www.ncbi.nlm.nih.gov/pubmed/17076983.

Birbrair, Alexander, et al. "Type-1 Pericytes Accumulate after Tissue Injury and Produce Collagen in an Organ-dependent Manner." *Stem Cell Research & Therapy* 5 (2014): 122. Accessed May 5, 2019. https://stemcellres. biomedcentral.com/articles/10.1186/scrt512.

Bober, Michael B, M.D. "Osteogenesis Imperfecta (Brittle Bone Disease)." KidsHealth. Accessed May 3, 2019. https://kidshealth.org/en/parents/ osteogenesis-imperfecta.html.

Borumand, Maryam, et al. "Effects of a nutritional supplement containing collagen peptides on skin elasticity, hydration and wrinkles." *Journal of Medical Nutrition & Nutraceuticals* 4, no. 1 (2015): 47–53. Accessed March 5, 2019. https://www.ncbi.nlm.nih.gov/books/NBK21582/.

Bruyere, O., et al. "Effect of Collagen Hydrolysate in Articular Pain: A 6-month Randomized, Double-blind, Placebo Controlled Study." *Complementary Theories in Medicine* 20, no. 3 (2012): 124–130. Accessed May 3, 2019. https://www.ncbi.nlm.nih.gov/pubmed/22500661.

Chen, P., et al. "Lack of Collagen VI Promotes Wound-Induced Hair Growth." *Journal of Investigative Dermatology* 135, no. 10 (2015): 2358–67, accessed May 8, 2019. https://www.ncbi.nlm.nih.gov/pubmed/25989472.

Choi, Franchesca D., et al. "Oral Collagen Supplementation: A Systematic Review of Dermatological Applications." *Journal of Drugs in Dermatology* 18, no. 1 (2019): 9–16. Accessed March 25, 2019. https://www.ncbi.nlm.nih. gov/pubmed/30681787.

Clark, K. L., et al. "24-Week Study on the Use of Collagen Hydrolysate as a Dietary Supplement in Athletes with Activity-Related Joint Pain." *Current Medical Research and Opinion* 24, no. 5 (2008): 1485–96. Accessed April 2, 2019. https://www.ncbi.nlm.nih.gov/pubmed/18416885.

Czajka, A., et al. "Daily Oral Supplementation with Collagen Peptides Combined with Vitamins and Other Bioactive Compounds Improves Skin Elasticity and Has a Beneficial Effect on Joint and General Wellbeing." *Nutrition Research* 57 (2018): 97–108. Accessed March 29, 2019. https:// www.ncbi.nlm.nih.gov/pubmed/30122200.

Dar, Qurratul-Ain, et al. "Daily Oral Consumption of Hydrolyzed Type 1 Collagen Is Chondroprotective and Anti-inflammatory in Murine Posttraumatic Osteoarthritis." *PLoS One* 12, no. 4 (2017): e0174705. Accessed March 25, 2019. https://www.ncbi.nlm.nih.gov/pmc/articles/ PMC5383229/.

de Almeida Jackix, E., et al. "A Food Supplement of Hydrolyzed Collagen Improves Compositional and Biodynamic Characteristics of Vertebrae in Ovariectomized Rats." *Journal of Medicinal Food* 13, no. 6 (2010): 1385–90. Accessed March 16, 2019. https://www.ncbi.nlm.nih.gov/pubmed/20874246.

De Luca, Chiara, et al. "Skin Antiageing and Systemic Redox Effects of Supplementation with Marine Collagen Peptides and Plant-Derived Antioxidants: A Single-Blind Case-Control Clinical Study." *Oxidative Medicine and Cellular Longevity* (2016): 4389410. Accessed May 4, 2019. https://www.ncbi.nlm.nih.gov/pmc/articles/PMC4745978/.

Elam, M. L., et al. "A calcium-collagen chelate dietary supplement attenuates bone loss in postmenopausal women with osteopenia: a randomized controlled trial." *Journal of Medicinal Food* 18, no. 3 (2015): 324–31. Accessed April 5, 2019. https://www.ncbi.nlm.nih.gov/pubmed/25314004.

Elliott, Brianna, RD. "Top 6 Benefits of Taking Collagen Supplements." Healthline. Accessed February 6, 2019. https://www.healthline.com/nutrition/collagen-benefits.

Eyre, D. "Collagen of articular cartilage." *Arthritis Research & Therapy* 4, no. 1 (2000): 30–5. Accessed April 4, 2019. https://www.ncbi.nlm.nih.gov/pubmed/11879535.

Ganceviciene, Ruta, et al. "Skin Anti-Aging Strategies." *DermatoEndicronology* 4, no. 3 (2012): 308–19. Accessed March 29, 2019. https://www.ncbi.nlm.nih.gov/pmc/articles/PMC3583892/.

Garcia-Coronado, J. M., et al. "Effect of Collagen Supplementation on Osteoarthritis Symptoms: A Meta-analysis of Randomized Placebo-Controlled Trials." *International Orthopaedics* 43, no. 3 (2019): 531–8. Accessed March 1, 2019. https://www.ncbi.nlm.nih.gov/pubmed/30368550.

Gillies, Allison R., et al. "Structure and Function of the Skeletal Muscle Extracellular Matrix." *Muscle & Nerve* 44, no. 3 (2011): 318-331. Accessed April 5, 2019. https://www.ncbi.nlm.nih.gov/pmc/articles/PMC3177172/.

Harris, E. D., et al. "Copper and the Synthesis of Elastin and Collagen." *Ciba Foundation Symposium* 79 (1980): 163–82. Accessed May 2, 2019. https://www.ncbi.nlm.nih.gov/pubmed/6110524.

Hays, N. P., et al. "Effects of whey and fortified collagen hydrolysate protein supplements on nitrogen balance and body composition in older women." *Journal of the Academy of Nutrition and Dietetics* 109, no. 6 (2009): 1082–7. Accessed March 29, 2019. https://www.ncbi.nlm.nih.gov/pubmed/19465192.

Hexsel, Doris, MD, et al. "Oral supplementation with specific bioactive collagen peptides improves nail growth and reduces symptoms of brittle nails." *Journal of Cosmetic Dermatology* 16, no. 4 (2017): 520–6. Accessed May 10, 2019. https://onlinelibrary.wiley.com/doi/abs/10.1111/jocd.12393.

Holmgren, Steven K., et al. "A Hyperstable Collagen Mimic." *Chemistry & Biology* 6 (1999): 63–70. Accessed May 1, 2019. https://www.cell.com/cell-chemical-biology/pdf/S1074-5521%2899%2980003-9.pdf.

Holzapfel, Gerhard A. "Biomechanics of Soft Tissue," *Handbook of Materials Behavior Models* 3 (2001): 1057–71. Accessed May 3, 2019. https://www.sciencedirect.com/science/article/pii/B9780124433410501071.

Hsu, Ching-Yun, et al. "The Antioxidant and Free Radical Scavenging Activities of Chlorophylls and Pheophytins." *Food and Nutrition Sciences* 4 (2013): 1–8. Accessed May 1, 2019. http://file.scirp.org/pdf/FNS_2013072614461013.pdf.

Ito, Naoki, et al. "Effects of Composite Supplement Containing Collagen Peptide and Ornithine on Skin Conditions and Plasma IGF-1 Levels—A Randomized, Double-Blind, Placebo-Controlled Trial." *Marine Drugs* 16, no. 12 (2018): 482. Accessed March 2, 2019. https://www.ncbi.nlm.nih.gov/pmc/articles/PMC6315531/.

Iwai, Koji, et al. "Identification of Food-Derived Collagen Peptides in Human Blood after Oral Ingestion of Gelatin Hydrolysates." *Journal of Agricultural and Food Chemistry* 53, no. 16 (2005): 6531–6. Accessed May 1, 2019. https://pubs.acs.org/doi/abs/10.1021/jf050206p.

Jennings, Kerri-Ann, MS, RD. "Collagen—What Is It and What Is It Good For?" Healthline. Accessed February 10, 2019. https://www.healthline.com/nutrition/collagen.

Kafi, R., et al. "Improvement of Naturally Aged Skin with Vitamin A (Retinol)." *Archives of Dermatology* 143, no. 5 (2007): 606–12. Accessed May 3, 2019. https://www.ncbi.nlm.nih.gov/pubmed/17515510.

Kim, H. K., et al. "Osteogenic Activity of Collagen Peptide Via ERK/MAPK Pathway Mediated Boosting of Collagen Synthesis and Its Therapeutic Efficacy in Osteoporotic Bone by Back-scattered Electron Imaging and Microarchitecture Analysis." *Molecules* 18, no. 12 (2013): 15474–89. Accessed April 3, 2019. https://www.ncbi.nlm.nih.gov/pubmed/24352008.

Kim, D. U., et al. "Oral Intake of Low-Molecular-Weight Collagen Peptide Improves Hydration, Elasticity, and Wrinkling in Human Skin: A Randomized, Double-Blind, Placebo-Controlled Study." *Nutrientis* 10, no. 7 (2018): 826. Accessed March 1, 2019. https://www.ncbi.nlm.nih.gov/pmc/articles/PMC6073484/.

Konig, Daniel, et al. "Specific Collagen Peptides Improve Bone Mineral Density and Bone Markers in Postmenopausal Women—A Randomized Controlled Study." *Nutrients* 10, no. 1 (2018): 97. Accessed March 1, 2019. https://www.ncbi.nlm.nih.gov/pmc/articles/PMC5793325/.

Koutroubakis, I. E., et al. "Serum Laminin and Collagen IV in Inflammatory Bowel Disease." *Journal of Clinical Pathology* 56, no. 11 (2003): 817–20. Accessed May 3, 2019. https://www.ncbi.nlm.nih.gov/pubmed/14600124.

Kumar, S., et al. "A Double-blind, Placebo-controlled, Randomised, Clinical Study on the Effectiveness of Collagen Peptide on Osteoarthritis." *Journal of the Science of Food and Agriculture* 95, no. 4 (2015): 702–7. Accessed March 2, 2019. https://www.ncbi.nlm.nih.gov/pubmed/24852756.

Letourneau, P. C. "Axonal Pathfinding: Extracellular Matrix Role," *Encyclopedia of Neuroscience* (2016). Accessed May 5, 2019. https://www.sciencedirect.com/science/article/pii/B9780128093245026304.

Link, Rachael, MS, RD. "Bone Marrow: Nutrition, Benefits, and Food Sources." Healthline. Accessed April 17, 2019. https://www.healthline.com/nutrition/bone-marrow.

Lodish, Harvey, et al. *Molecular Cell Biology*, 4th edition (2000).

Mayo Clinic Staff. "Stop Smoking." Mayo Clinic. Accessed May 7, 2019. https://www.mayoclinic.org/es-es/healthy-lifestyle/quit-smoking/expert-answers/smoking/faq-20058153.

McIntosh, James. "Collagen: What Is It and What Are Its Uses?" Medical News Today. Accessed February 10, 2019. https://www.medicalnewstoday.com/articles/262881.php.

Michels, Alexander J., PhD. "Vitamin C and Skin Health." Oregon State University. Accessed May 3, 2019. https://lpi.oregonstate.edu/mic/health-disease/skin-health/vitamin-C.

Michels, Alexander J., PhD. "Vitamin E and Skin Health." Oregon State University. Accessed May 3, 2019. https://lpi.oregonstate.edu/mic/health-disease/skin-health/vitamin-E.

Moskowitz, R. W. "Role of collagen hydrolysate in bone and joint disease." *Seminars in Arthritis and Rheumatism* 30, no. 2 (2000): 87–99. Accessed April 2, 2019. https://www.ncbi.nlm.nih.gov/pubmed/11071580.

Murakami, Hitoshi, et al. "Importance of Amino Acid Composition to Improve Skin Collagen Protein Synthesis Rates in UV-irradiated Mice." *Amino Acids* 42, no. 6 (2012): 2481–9. Accessed May 6, 2019. https://www.ncbi.nlm.nih.gov/pmc/articles/PMC3351609/.

Nandhini, A. T., et al. "Taurine Prevents Collagen Abnormalities in High Fructose-fed Rats." *Indian Journal of Medical Research* 122, no. 2 (2005): 171–7. Accessed May 4, 2019. https://www.ncbi.nlm.nih.gov/pubmed/16177476.

Oesser, S., et al. "Stimulation of Type II Collagen Biosynthesis and Secretion in Bovine Chondrocytes Cultured with Degraded Collagen." *Cell and Tissue Research* 311, no. 3 (2003): 393–9. Accessed March 16, 2019. https://www.ncbi.nlm.nih.gov/pubmed/12658447.

Porfirio, Elisangela, et al. "Collagen supplementation as a complementary therapy for the prevention and treatment of osteoporosis and osteoarthritis: a systematic review." *Revista Brasileira de Geriatria e Gerontologia* 19, no. 1 (2016): 153–64. Accessed March 29, 2019. http://www.scielo.br/pdf/rbgg/v19n1/1809-9823-rbgg-19-01-00153.pdf.

Proksch, E., et al. "Oral Supplementation of Specific Collagen Peptides Has Beneficial Effects on Human Skin Physiology: A Double-blind, Placebo-controlled Study." *Skin Pharmacology and Physiology*, 27, no. 1 (2014): 47–55. Accessed March 25, 2019. https://www.ncbi.nlm.nih.gov/pubmed/23949208.

Pullar, Juliet M., et al. "The Roles of Vitamin C in Skin Health." *Nutrients* 9, no. 8 (2017): 866. Accessed May 3, 2019. https://www.ncbi.nlm.nih.gov/pmc/articles/PMC5579659/.

Rutter, Kathryn, et al. "Green Tea Extract Suppresses the Age-Related Increase in Collagen Crosslinking and Fluorescent Products in C57BL/6 Mice." *International Journal for Vitamin and Nutrition Research* 73, no. 6 (2003): 453–60. Accessed May 3, 2019. https://www.ncbi.nlm.nih.gov/pmc/articles/PMC3561737/.

Schauss, A. G., et al. "Effect of the novel low molecular weight hydrolyzed chicken sternal cartilage extract, BioCell Collagen, on improving osteoarthritis-related symptoms: a randomized, double-blind, placebo-controlled trial." *Journal of Agricultural and Food Chemistry* 25, no. 60 (2012): 4096–101. Accessed April 2, 2019. https://www.ncbi.nlm.nih.gov/pubmed/22486722.

Schunck, Michael, et al. "Dietary Supplementation with Specific Collagen Peptides Has a Body Mass Index-Dependent Beneficial Effect on Cellulite Morphology." *Journal of Medicinal Food* 18, no. 12 (2015): 1340–8. Accessed May 1, 2019. https://www.ncbi.nlm.nih.gov/pmc/articles/PMC4685482/.

Schwartz, Stephen R., et al. "Ingestion of BioCell Collagen®, a Novel Hydrolyzed Chicken Sternal Cartilage Extract; Enhanced Blood Microcirculation and Reduced Facial Aging Signs." *Clinical Interventions in Aging* 7 (2012): 267–73. Accessed May 3, 2019. https://www.ncbi.nlm.nih.gov/pmc/articles/PMC3426261/.

Seo, Hyun-Ju, et al. "Zinc May Increase Bone Formation Through Stimulating Cell Proliferation, Alkaline Phosphatase Activity and Collagen Synthesis in Osteoblastic MC3T3-E1 Cells." *Nutrition Research and Practice* 4, no. 5. (2010): 356–61. Accessed May 2, 2019. https://synapse.koreamed.org/DOIx.php?id=10.4162/nrp.2010.4.5.356.

Shoulders, Matthew D. "Collagen Structure and Stability," *Annual Review of Biochemistry* 78 (2009): 929–58. Accessed May 1, 2019. https://www.ncbi.nlm.nih.gov/pmc/articles/PMC2846778/.

Song, Hongdong, et al. "Effect of Orally Administered Collagen Peptides from Bovine Bone on Skin Aging in Chronologically Aged Mice." *Nutrients* 9, no. 11 (2017): 1209. Accessed March 26, 2019. https://www.ncbi.nlm.nih.gov/pmc/articles/PMC5707681/.

Sripriya, Ramasamy, et al. "A Novel Enzymatic Method for Preparation and Characterization of Collagen Film from Swim Bladder of Fish Rohu (Labeo rohita)." *Food and Nutrition Sciences* 6, no. 15 (2015): 1468–78. Accessed May 3, 2019. https://www.ncbi.nlm.nih.gov/books/NBK21582/.

Stevens, Cara J. "Is Hydrolyzed Collagen a Miracle Cure?" Healthline. Accessed March 4, 2019. https://www.healthline.com/health/food-nutrition/is-hydrolyzed-collagen-a-miracle-cure.

Strawbridge, Holly. "Artificial Sweeteners: Sugar-free, But at What Cost?" Harvard Health Publishing. Accessed May 5, 2019. https://www.health.harvard.edu/blog/artificial-sweeteners-sugar-free-but-at-what-cost-201207165030.

Takeda, Satoko, et al. "Hydrolyzed Collagen Intake Increases Bone Mass of Growing Rats Trained with Running Exercise." *Journal of the International Society of Sports Nutrition* 10 (2013): 35. Accessed March 15, 2019. https://www.ncbi.nlm.nih.gov/pmc/articles/PMC3750261/.

Telang, Pumori Saokar. "Vitamin C in Dermatology." *Indian Dermatology Online Journal* 4, no. 2 (2013): 143–6. Accessed May 2, 2019. http://www.idoj.in/article.asp?issn=2229-5178;year=2013;volume=4;issue=2;spage=143;epage=146;aulast=Telang.

Tengrup, I., et al. "Influence of zinc on synthesis and the accumulation of collagen in early granulation tissue." *Surgery, Gynecology & Obstetrics* 153, no. 3 (1981): 323–6. Accessed May 2, 2019. https://www.ncbi.nlm.nih.gov/pubmed/7466582.

Tomosugi, Naohisa, et al. "Effect of Collagen Tripeptide on Atherosclerosis in Healthy Humans." *Journal of Atherosclerosis and Thrombosis* 24, no. 5 (2017): 530–8. Accessed May 1, 2019. https://www.ncbi.nlm.nih.gov/pmc/articles/PMC5429168/.

Traber, Maret G., et al. "Vitamins C and E: Beneficial Effects from a Mechanistic Perspective." *Free Radical Biology and Medicine* 51, no. 5 (2011): 1000–13. Accessed May 2, 2019. https://www.sciencedirect.com/science/article/pii/S0891584911003194?via%3Dihub.

Trookman, Nathan S., et al. "Immediate and Long-term Clinical Benefits of a Topical Treatment for Facial Lines and Wrinkles." *The Journal of Clinical and Aesthetic Dermatology* 2, no. 3 (2009): 38–43. Accessed March 3, 2019. https://www.ncbi.nlm.nih.gov/pmc/articles/PMC2923951/.

Van De Walle, Gavin, MS, RD. "Top 9 Benefits and Uses of Glycine." Healthline. Accessed May 2, 2019. https://www.healthline.com/nutrition/glycine.

Varani, James, et al. "Vitamin A Antagonizes Decreased Cell Growth and Elevated Collagen-Degrading Matrix Metalloproteinases and Stimulates Collagen Accumulation in Naturally Aged Human Skin." *Journal of Investigative Dermatology* 114, no. 3 (2000): 480–6. Accessed March 6, 2019. https://www.ncbi.nlm.nih.gov/pubmed/10692106/.

Watson, Kathryn. "5 Ways to Boost Collagen." Healthline. Accessed February 5, 2019. https://www.healthline.com/health/ways-to-boost-collagen.

Zdzieblik, Denise, et al. "Collagen Peptide Supplementation in Combination with Resistance Training Improves Body Composition and Increases Muscle Strength in Elderly Sarcopenic Men: A Randomised Controlled Trial." *The British Journal of Nutrition* 114, no. 8 (2015): 1237–45. Accessed May 1, 2019. https://www.ncbi.nlm.nih.gov/pmc/articles/PMC4594048/.

Zhu, C.F., et al. "Therapeutic Effects of Marine Collagen Peptides on Chinese Patients with Type 2 Diabetes Mellitus and Primary Hypertension." *The American Journal of the Medical Sciences* 340, no. 6 (2010): 360–6. Accessed March 1, 2019. https://www.ncbi.nlm.nih.gov/pubmed/20739874.

INDEX

IMAGE CREDITS

ACKNOWLEDGMENTS

This book is the culmination of more than a decade's worth of professional investment by people I've been so fortunate to meet as our paths crossed. I am better because of every manager, editor, writer, and friend I've made from the start of my career to today.

Thank you to my parents, who were the biggest fans of my first published work, a third-grade news magazine about animals in rainforests, as well as every work since then. They never batted an eye when I tried out one college program after another, and likewise didn't falter when I decided to quit my job for the great unknown of freelance writing. It seems my curious nature and tendency to explore were rooted at an early age. That inquisitiveness is key for a journalist!

Thank you to my journalism professors at Samford University in Birmingham, Alabama, who saw a determined, if not always organized and ordered, young woman and encouraged me every step of the way, even long after graduation day.

Thank you to my friends who were willing to give honest feedback on a tricky paragraph, who share with joy the stories I write, and who keep me grounded when deadlines seem near to doing me in.

Thank you also to my editors, Nicole Fisher and Jennifer Williams, for shepherding me through this experience. I am thankful for your patience and wisdom. Thank you also to the Sterling Publishing team for putting together such a fun and captivating book.

This book is also only possible because of a lifetime of support from my family. Thank you for encouraging me, checking in, and occasionally sending spicy tuna rolls to make sure I remembered to eat while filing this book and so many other projects.

ABOUT THE AUTHOR

KIMBERLY HOLLAND is a food, lifestyle, and health writer. For Holland, food is both a joy and a way of caring for yourself and others. The former editor of CookingLight.com and current senior editor of Allrecipes.com, Kimberly's work has also been featured in various print and online publications, including *EatingWell*, *Real Simple*, *Southern Living*, and Healthline, among others.

CAROLYN WILLIAMS, PhD, RD, a James Beard Award-winning dietitian and culinary nutrition expert, is dedicated to serving media, lifestyle brands, and health professionals with accurate and consumer-friendly solutions. Williams develops content for various media outlets and lifestyle brands such as *Real Simple*, *Parents*, *EatingWell*, *eMeals*, and *Health*. She is the author of *Meals That Heal*, which focuses on the healing aspects of food.